T0194910

THE
KEY TO
HEALTHY
LIVING

A COVID-19
Warrior
Talks About
Health

THE KEY TO HEALTHY LIVING

A COVID-19
Warrior
Talks About
Health

Zhong Nanshan

Guangzhou Institute of Respiratory Diseases, China

Translated by

John Qiong Wang

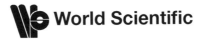

World Scientific

NEW JERSEY · LONDON · SINGAPORE · BEIJING · SHANGHAI · HONG KONG · TAIPEI · CHENNAI · TOKYO

Published by

World Scientific Publishing Co. Pte. Ltd.

5 Toh Tuck Link, Singapore 596224

USA office: 27 Warren Street, Suite 401-402, Hackensack, NJ 07601

UK office: 57 Shelton Street, Covent Garden, London WC2H 9HE

British Library Cataloguing-in-Publication Data
A catalogue record for this book is available from the British Library.

《钟南山谈健康》
Originally published in Chinese by Guangdong Education Publishing House Co. Ltd.
Copyright © Guangdong Education Publishing House Co. Ltd. 2020

THE KEY TO HEALTHY LIVING
A COVID-19 Warrior Talks About Health

ISBN 978-981-123-680-8 (hardcover)
ISBN 978-981-123-748-5 (paperback)
ISBN 978-981-123-681-5 (ebook for institutions)
ISBN 978-981-123-682-2 (ebook for individuals)

For any available supplementary material, please visit
https://www.worldscientific.com/worldscibooks/10.1142/12272#t=suppl

Typeset by Stallion Press
Email: enquiries@stallionpress.com

Printed in Singapore

Foreword

by Guangdong Education Publishing House

Upon the melting of ice and snow, the cold winter leaves quietly and we welcome the arrival of a warm spring. At this moment, we may forget everything, but what we will never forget is the breath-taking battle against SARS in 2003, which was a war without smoke. For victory, we salute to each other; for history, we shall remember it forever!

Many in China know and admire Zhong Nanshan, an academician of the Chinese Academy of Engineering, a former president of the Chinese Medical Association, and a great doctor listed in "Touching China[1]". He was a leader in the battle against SARS and has made key contributions to the epidemic control. It was he who pointed out in a scientific manner that SARS was "preventable, treatable and controllable" when the public was in a state of panic during the early days of SARS. It was he who shouted loudly "we volunteer to treat the most severe patients" with a heroic attitude of facing death unflinchingly. It was he who led the team to develop effective treatment plans. It was he who advocated international scientific and technological cooperation to deal with the common epidemic of all mankind, despite facing criticism.

---

[1] The annual "Touching China" program, which was first broadcast in 2003, honors those who have touched the nation with their tenacity, bravery and wisdom over the previous year.

"The key factor to a well-off society is health." After the battle against SARS, Dr. Zhong Nanshan, despite his workload, continues to care about the physical and mental health of the Chinese people. He proposed to the national leaders and authorities that "young citizens have stature but lack physical fitness. This is so worrying." He also submitted other proposals for healthcare reform at the National People's Congress (NPC) and Chinese People's Political Consultative Conference (CPPCC), garnering extensive social attention. When the COVID-19 epidemic began in 2020, 84-year-old Zhong Nanshan, together with other scientists and medical workers, directly fought against the epidemic. Every single day, we continue to be touched by their contributions. When people didn't care about the epidemic in the beginning, Dr. Zhong warned that "it is for sure that inter-person transmission of the novel coronavirus pneumonia exists and it is likely that the virus originated from wild animals" and "10 to 14 days is a reasonable isolation and observation period. After the incubation period, people who are sick should receive treatment in time, while those who show no symptoms are free from infection of COVID-19." We feel particularly relieved as truth can convince the entire world in this case. During this epidemic, we especially trust Dr. Zhong. He is also an enthusiastic disseminator of health concepts. He has been frequently invited by governments of all levels, enterprises and institutions to give lectures and has received great attention and responses. Dr. Zhong has talked about health, sub-health, decisive factors affecting human health and the cornerstone of human health in an era of rapid changes and fierce competition from a scientific point of view. His words are sincere and convincing.

Dr. Zhong has proposed many new health concepts. For instance,

"Health is like a hollow glass ball, once it falls to the ground, it will be shattered and there will be nothing left. Work is like a rubber ball, which can rebound after falling down."

"Life is limited and health is priceless."

"Health is a one-way street and we can only advance."

"We should learn to care about our own health."

"We should carry out early prevention and treatment, and minor injuries should be taken seriously."

"Your lifestyle for 20 years determines your body 20 years later."

He also proposed some viable self-care and self-examination approaches. Feedback from listeners is that Dr. Zhong's lectures and talks are like the spring breeze and the knowledge gleaned has freed them from various health issues that have worried them for years.

Dr. Zhong summarized the five cornerstones of health: psychological balance, reasonable diet, no smoking and limited alcohol, sufficient exercise, early prevention and treatment. He paid great attention to early prevention and treatment. Indeed, Dr. Zhong has demonstrated that the top 10 diseases in China (e.g., tumors, high blood pressure, diabetes mellitus, coronary disease, chronic obstructive pulmonary disease) can be identified via some small symptoms before development into fatal problems such as myocardial infarction and cerebrovascular accident after 5, 10 or even 15 years. Many young and middle-aged people think that they are young and in good health. Usually, they tend to ignore abnormal physical conditions and will not go to the hospital until the problem is severe, resulting in irreparable losses and even death in extreme cases.

Dr. Zhong believes that early prevention and treatment achieves a big return on a small investment. Generally, seniors tend to pay attention to health. If they can do it 20 to 30 years earlier and prevention has been considered when they are in good health, a maximum return can be achieved with minimum investment. Dr. Zhong has introduced that the development of health education activities in clinical work to provide self-management information for asthma patients in hospitals and equip patients with self-management techniques. As a result, the recurrence rate of asthma was reduced by 75% and the hospitalization time was reduced by 54%, resulting in a greatly reduced economic and psychological burden for patients.

Dr. Zhong emphasized that the unhealthiest 1% of the population and those suffering from chronic diseases (19% of the population) account for 70% of total healthcare expenses, while 70% of the healthy population account for only 10% of total healthcare expenses.

It is impossible for anyone to be healthy forever and anyone may become one of the unhealthiest 1% or the 19% suffering from chronic diseases in the future. However, we must bear in mind Dr. Zhong's advice that "my health is in my own hands" and conduct regular inspections to achieve early detection, early diagnosis and early treatment so that any disease can be controlled in its infancy. Such measures can not only greatly reduce the chance of illness and the pain of individuals, but also effectively prolong the lifespan of the citizens, thus conserving national resources. Therefore, Dr. Zhong's efforts in preventive medicine and popular science are of great significance to the country and the public.

Dr. Zhong's seminars were wonderful and vivid, and highly beneficial to the audience. Indeed, the content of his seminars have spread widely all over China. Aims to collaborate with Dr. Zhong in promotion of preventive medicine and popularization of scientific health concepts, the Guangdong Education Publishing House published Dr. Zhong's first book on health-care after thorough discussions with him.

This book was written by Dr. Zhong based on his lectures and seminars. For the convenience of readers, it has been divided into Sections A, B and C with sub-headings. Alongside the lively illustrations and datasets, the main-points are summarized at the beginning of each section.

It is indeed our honor to collaborate with Dr. Zhong in order to pro-mote preventive medicine and popularize scientific health concepts. It is our hope that this book will make a contribution to the health of readers and the prosperity of our country.

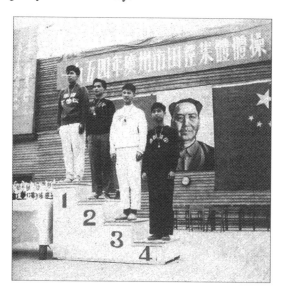

In 1954, Dr. Zhong Nanshan was ranked 4th in the track and field competition in Guangzhou.

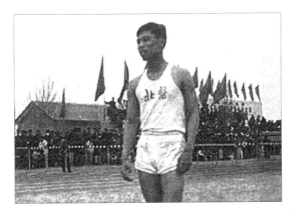

In 1960, Dr. Zhong Nanshan as a competitive sportsman and student at Beijing Medical College.

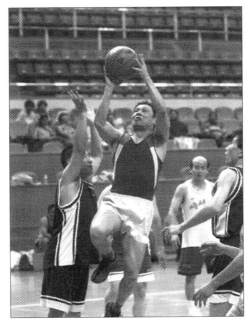

Dr. Zhong Nanshan playing basketball (during the fight against SARS in 2003).

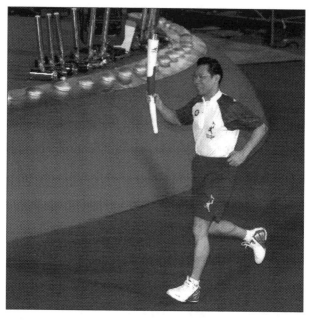

In October 25, 2006, the torch of the Doha Asian Games arrived in Guangzhou. Dr. Zhong Nanshan was the last runner in the torch relay.

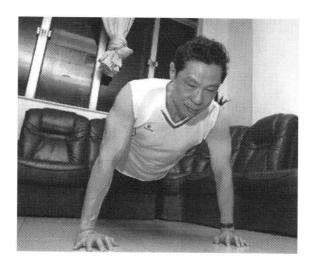

In 2009, 73-year-old Zhong Nanshan doing push-ups at home.

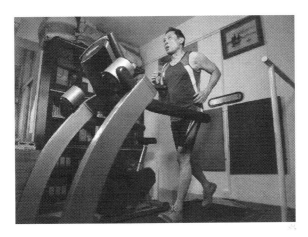

In 2018, 82-year-old Zhong Nanshan running in a family gym.

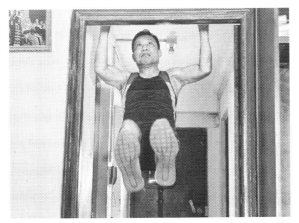

In 2018, 82-year-old Zhong Nanshan doing pull-ups at home.

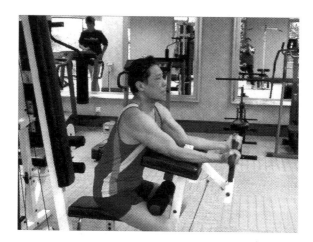

Dr. Zhong Nanshan working out at the gym.

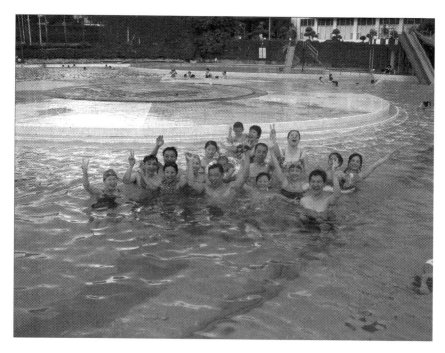

Dr. Zhong Nanshan swimming with his colleagues.

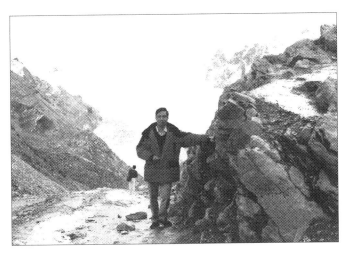

Dr. Zhong Nanshan goes hiking.

Contents

Section A

About Health

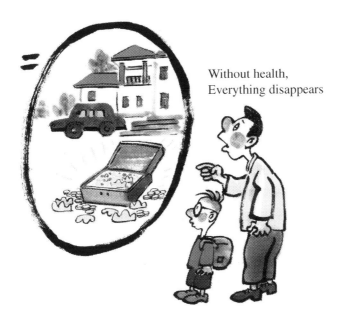

Without health,
Everything disappears

"Health does not guarantee everything, but health is the foundation of everything."

We live in an era with rapid change and fierce competition and this era provides good opportunities for those who are willing to work for a better life. We are all fighting for achievements and new peaks in our lives, which, however, repeatedly challenge the limits of our body. Unfortunately, some of us "advance" too much from the health "bank", resulting in illness or even early death.

The 21st century is a century of longevity. American scholars suggest that by 2080, the average age of the global population can reach 97 years and the average age of women can reach 100 years. In 1999, the former UN Secretary General Kofi Annan declared to the world on the International Day of Older Persons that "everyone can enjoy 100 years." There is an old Chinese saying that "people smile happily at the age of 100, 90 years old is not rare, 80 years old is common, 70 years old is young and 60 years old is infancy." At the age of 60, a person is halfway on his/her life journey and shall meet challenges again. From this point of view, the old proverb "70 years old is rare" is no longer valid. What is the basis of longevity? It is health. Only health can lead to longevity. Hong Zhaoguang, a well-known healthcare education expert, has an impressive saying:

> "Health and happiness can lead to the age of 100 years if we are in good mood every day; if we do not get sick before 60 years old, we can keep healthy until retirement, and we will not age before 80 years old, thus reaching 100 years old easily; staying healthy can have advantages such as less suffering for oneself, reduced burden for children, saving on medical expenses and benefiting the society."

I believe we all share the wish of being healthy, enjoying life and doing whatever we want. Everyone in the world has fortune, whether large or small. I believe health should be the first and most valuable fortune. Without health, other fortunes make no sense. Madame Curie said that the foundation of science is health. Anyone ignoring health is joking with his/her life.

Health is the foundation of the future

"Sometimes death is not a sad thing, for at least the dead can take a rest forever..." If someone expresses such a view on life and death, can you guess his occupation? This is a comment an employee of an IT (Information Technology) enterprise left in response to the death of Jan Malm, the former president of Ericsson (China) Communications Co., Ltd, on an Internet forum. This is more than a complaint or escapist statement, in fact, it is a sort of self-criticism.

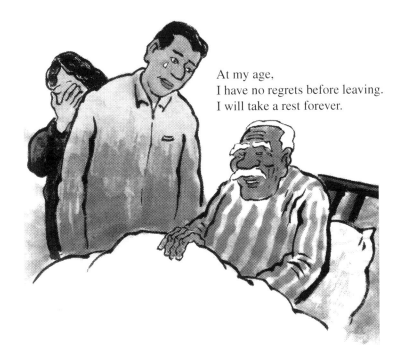

At my age,
I have no regrets before leaving.
I will take a rest forever.

On the evening of April 8, 2004, Jan Malm, who had the habit of exercising, went to the gym. He had been occupied by work and postponed exercise several times due to a business trip to Shanghai. Unfortunately, he did not expect that he would have to pay the price of life. After days of overloaded and intense work, his heart could no longer bear the intensive exercise. While running on the treadmill, his heart stopped beating suddenly. The Swedish man, who "spent all his time working", collapsed without exhibiting any signs of illness at the age of 54 years old.

Let's take a look at the life of Zhang, a technical engineer working for a well-known international communications company: the working hours are from 9:00 a.m. to 2:00 a.m. the next day, with a break of only two hours for eating and commuting. Sometimes he has to work even after returning home. Zhang feels sick and has no time for exercise. Nevertheless, he has no choice because both the company and himself are under great pressure: the company is facing fierce competition and the employees have KPIs (Key Performance Indicators) to meet. Anyone who doesn't work hard can be replaced at any time. Therefore, every nerve in Zhang's body is tense. Zhang did not comment too much on Jan Malm's death.

He claimed that anyone choosing this job should have expected such an outcome. In this era of competition, anyone who doesn't work hard will be replaced. "He said he was still young and his body could bear it."

I have noticed the comments on Jan Malm's death online. Many people feel sorry and express dissatisfaction with the current situation. However, few try to change the current situation. Everyone thinks that employees should work hard and that working overtime is natural.

As I acknowledged earlier, our current era of rapid change and fierce competition provides us myraid opportunities for work and advancement in life. This is positive development. But it becomes negative when one challenges the limits of body again and again for work as it is very dangerous. Some people "advance" too much from their health "banks", resulting in severe sickness and even early death. This is a tragedy that should be avoided. I hope everyone realizes this fact as soon as possible, attach importance to healthcare, and take good care of their bodies. With physical and psychological health, we can plant the seedlings of "fortune" and sow the seeds of "career" on the "green hill" of health. Then, we cultivate thoroughly to achieve a successful life.

An acute disease alarmed me

I believe in an old saying: "Good fortune follows upon disaster, disaster lurks within good fortune." It means that we should learn to look at both sides of frustrations in life. I have a deep understanding and personal experience of this. Before my wakeup call, I believed I was in good health. During the fight against SARS in 2003, our hospital admitted many severe cases. SARS was an entirely new disease and there were no precedent cases for references. At that time, we worked day and night to find an effective treatment. As a result, I felt that my body was a bit overworked, but I didn't pay too much attention to it. Later, the SARS epidemic was brought under control and we were supposed to take a rest. Nevertheless, I did not stop working as I thought I had a "good foundation." On August 23, 2004, I returned from a business trip to Beijing. During my stay in Beijing, I worked until 1:00 a.m. every day due to preparation for conferences and communications with others. When I returned to Guangzhou, I was so tired, but some students invited me to play badminton.

I could not refuse and played three games in succession. I felt exhausted. In the middle of the night, I suddenly felt the discomfort of the heart (chest oppression and respiratory distress) but I still did not go to the hospital until dawn. Inspection showed that my heart had suffered minor myocardial infarction (tissue death due to inadequate blood supply). Fortunately, cardiac stenting was arranged for me and I recovered soon afterwards.

This event severely lowered my confidence. I was so depressed and pessimistic. I started to feel that my body was not as good as before. One day, while I was walking, my cousin, who was working in Shanghai, called me. The first thing he said was, "Congratulations! You are so lucky." I was a bit unhappy when I heard this. Why did he congratulate me when I was so unlucky? He continued, "I congratulate you for three reasons. First, this event didn't happen on business trips, especially not abroad, so you could go to the hospital in time. Second, the infarction involved a small blood vessel instead of any important part. Third, this incident serves as a warning: pay attention to your health!" His words cheered me up. Without this accident, I would probably have continued eating fried and greasy things and not taken breaks from work. As a result, I would have been exposed to severe diseases or even death. Now, I have corrected many bad habits. Doesn't this show that a bad event can turn into a good thing?

Definition of health

It is well-known that health is very important, but what indeed is health? Well, there are a thousand Hamlets in a thousand people's eyes. Some believe that health means being free from sickness, while others believe that health means a well-functioning body. Some even claim that health comes after you've spent all your money! It has been proposed that the five conditions for health are "eating fast, walking fast, pooping fast, talking fast and falling asleep fast." In other words, a person with a good appetite, good muscle function, good digestive ability, good nervous system, and good communications capability is considered to be healthy. Some dictionaries define health as the "proper functioning of all tissues in the body and being free from diseases."

All of these statements are correct in some way, but cannot summarize the definition of health. Modern medicine claims that health includes not only disease-free conditions, normal anatomical and physiological functions but also proper personality, normal psychological condition, integrated social adaptability and harmonious interpersonal relationships. This makes absolute sense. It is hard to define a person who is not sick, but unhappy all day or unsociable as healthy. Hence, it is not easy to achieve real health, which requires an understanding of daily healthcare, frequent physical exercise, positive personality and proper psychological condition. Only with all these achieved, can one be considered healthy.

Let us also consider the definition by the World Health Organization (WHO) which I fully agree with:

1. Having sufficient energy to handle the pressures of daily life and work without feeling too nervous.
2. Being optimistic and positive, willing to take responsibility, not picky.
3. Be able to rest and sleeping well.
4. Strong adaptability to changes in the external environment.
5. Being able to resist common colds and infectious diseases.
6. Weight is appropriate, body is symmetrical, head, shoulder and hip positions are coordinated when standing.
7. Bright eyes, sharp reaction, eyelids are not swollen.
8. Clean teeth, no cavities, no pain, normal gum color and no bleeding.
9. Hair is shiny, no dandruff.
10. Muscles and skin are elastic.

In summary, the WHO proposed that human health includes four aspects: physical health, mental health, strong social adaptability and moral integrity.

Understanding sub-health

In my clinical work, I often encounter patients who frequently feel exhausted, have poor attention spans, degraded memory and slight

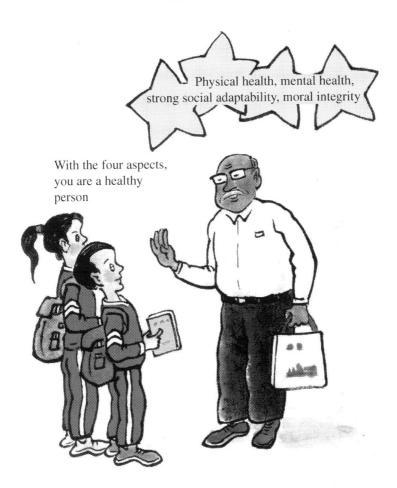

depression. However, medical examination suggest no abnormalities. They are so confused about that. In fact, these symptoms are that of sub-health.

WHO defines health as a state of complete physical, mental and social well-being, instead of physical strength alone or the absence of diseases. When this perfect balance is disrupted, the person is in a "sub-health" state. Sub-health reflects people's maladjustment in the physical, psychological and social aspect, and is a critical state between health and sickness. Generally, we may feel a sense of malaise or discomfort, but medical examination reveals nothing wrong. Studies show that only 15% of the total population meets the health standards in modern society. Interestingly, 15% of the total population is sick and unhealthy. If health and disease are regarded as its two ends, life is like an olive with two sharp ends and a convex middle part. The middle part is sub-health, which is a transitional state between health and sickness. Also, I would like to point out that at least 10% of the total population is between pre-sickness and sickness, which can be called a pre-clinical state. The pre-clinical state is one where the disease exists, but the symptoms are not obvious or have not attracted enough attention, or when the diagnosis is not yet definite. Strictly speaking, this group of people are already in an unhealthy state with diseases instead of sub-health. Therefore, this group shall be excluded from the sub-health group. In this case, the sub-health group accounts for 60% of the total population. Many people in the sub-health group believe that they are healthy. In fact, however, they cannot bear pressures from work and life as easily as healthy people do. Therefore, a correct understanding of sub-health and the driving factors of sub-health is a prerequisite for the prevention and treatment of sub-health.

Sub-health can be attributed to many factors, which can be judged according to the symptoms:

1. Mental stress and anxiety.
2. Loneliness, low self-esteem, melancholy and depression.
3. Dispersed attention and fickle-minded.
4. Frequent fury and unfounded worry.
5. Memory block and forgetting of acquaintances' names.
6. Fading interest and reduced desire for anything.
7. Limited communication and depression.
8. Easy exhaustion and eye pains.
9. Declined energy and slow movement.
10. Dizziness and slow recovery.
11. Dizziness after standing for a long time.
12. Soft limbs and poor strength.
13. Weight loss and physical weakness.
14. Difficulties in falling asleep and frequent dreaming.
15. Difficulties in getting up in the morning and frequent naps in the day.
16. Local numbness and cold hands and feet.
17. Sweaty palms and armpits, dry tongue and mouth.
18. Slight fever and night sweating.
19. Waist soreness followed by backache.

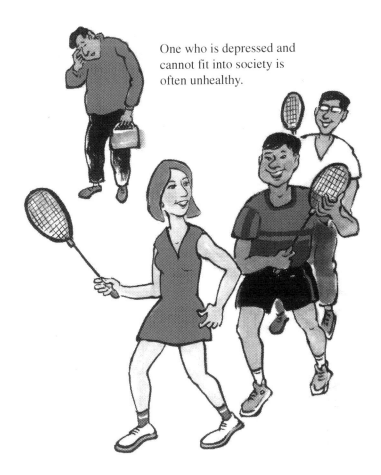

One who is depressed and cannot fit into society is often unhealthy.

20. White coating on the tongue and halitosic (chronic bad breath).
21. Repeated mouth and tongue ulcers.
22. Poor taste and appetite.
23. Acid regurgitation, belching, indigestion.
24. Constipation, abdominal fullness.
25. Frequent colds and herpes on lips.
26. Nasal congestion, runny nose, sore throat.
27. Shortness of breath.
28. Chest pain, chest oppression, cardiac pressure.
29. Palpitations and arrhythmia (irregular/abnormal heartbeat).
30. Tinnitus (ringing/noises in the ear) and slight deafness, carsickness.

... ...

I would like to remind readers that anyone feeling uncomfortable (exhausted, irritable, anxious, depressed) in your daily life frequently may be in sub-health.

Most white-collar workers are in the state of sub-health

There are a large number of people in the state of sub-health in our country, especially white-collar or "gold-collar" workers with "high education, high income and high pressure." Indeed, the growing rate of the sub-health group in China has surpassed those of developed countries in Europe and America. Herein, I would like to present statistical data to allow readers to develop an intuitive concept of the sub-health situation in China. In 2002, China Health Science and Technology Association collected statistics on sub-health in 14 provinces of China:

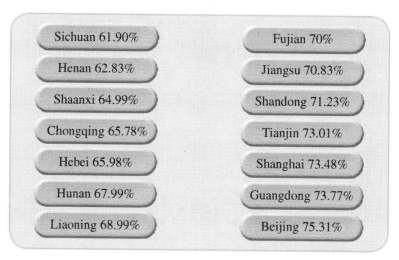

Sichuan 61.90%   Fujian 70%

Henan 62.83%   Jiangsu 70.83%

Shaanxi 64.99%   Shandong 71.23%

Chongqing 65.78%   Tianjin 73.01%

Hebei 65.98%   Shanghai 73.48%

Hunan 67.99%   Guangdong 73.77%

Liaoning 68.99%   Beijing 75.31%

The results of physical examination of 120,000 white-collar workers by a health examination center in Beijing (October 2004) are as follows:

As observed, most white-collar workers and entrepreneurs with "three highs" are in sub-health. Also, Beijing has the highest percentage of people of sub-health, followed by Guangzhou and Shanghai. These three places are the most economically developed areas in China. People in these cities face intense competition and the pressures of a fast-paced environment.

The sub-health situation in the education industry is not optimistic either. According to statistics, the ratio of sub-health in university

Table 1:   Physical examination results for white-collar workers.

Physical condition	Percentage of sample
At least one abnormal index (not specific)	89%
Hyperlipidemia (high levels of cholesterol)	27.89%
Fatty liver	26.61%
Hypertension (high blood pressure)	14.47%
Diabetes	5.88%
Abnormal electrocardiogram	9.43%
Gynecological diseases	12.35%
Tumor	50 persons/100,000
Chronic fatigue syndrome	35.23%
Sub-health state	69.53%

Table 2:   Survey on health status of Chinese entrepreneurs.

Physical condition	Percentage of sample
Gastrointestinal diseases	30.77%
Hyperglycemia (high blood sugar), high blood pressure, hyperlipidemia	23.08%
Excessive smoking and drinking	21.15%
Chronic fatigue	90.6%
Memory decline	28.3%
Insomnia	26.4%

teachers is 69.18% in China. Indeed, the ratio of university teachers aged 30–40 is up to 79.17%. In addition, the ratio of severe sub-health in females is significantly higher than in males. The main inducing factors include work pressure, psychological factors and inappropriate behaviors and habits. 44.21% of the participants were in moderate sub-health and

36.84% of the participants claimed sub-health. The survey also showed that the ratio of sub-health of teachers is higher than that of administrative and other personnel. To make it worse, there is a tendency of occupational diseases. For example, 70.29% of teachers had different degrees of sore throat, 80.15% of them felt neck pain, and 79.23% of them suffer from back pain, leg numbness and swelling. In other words, fatigue, which is commonly observed in university teachers, is a typical symptom of sub-health. As a veteran on the education front, I feel so worried about this situation.

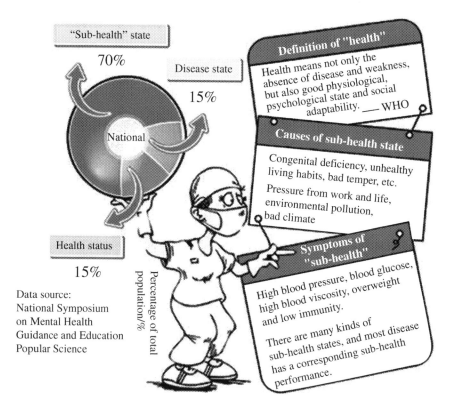

The ratio of sub-healthy people in China has reached 70%.

We all have three ages

As early as in the era of the Three Kingdoms, Cao Cao claimed "My destiny is governed by me not God." With the rapid development of science and technology, this is highly possible. We can get rid of the problem of age and actively take the initiative to delay aging. I am 84 years old this year, but many people who meet me for the first time don't believe it. They think I look much younger than my real age. I am very proud of this. I am 84 years old in biological age, 40 years old in physical age and 30 years old in mental age. Herein, there are three kinds of age involved.

The three ages of human beings refer to natural age, physiological age and psychological age. The natural age is our actual age (84 years old for me). The physiological age refers to the age reflected by body functions and appearances during the process of natural evolution. Some middle-aged people are exposed to signs of overall aging: white hair, wrinkles and poor physiological condition. They look like people in their sixties and seventies. In this case, their physiological age is defined to be sixties and seventies. On the contrary, some people are over 50 years old, but are ruddy-faced and look young. In this case, their physiological ages are below their actual ages. The psychological age is determined according to the degree of psychological aging, that is, whether a person has a healthy mentality. People of the same actual age may have significant differences in physical and psychological ages. A positive mentality will in turn reduce physical age. Elderly people may also have big ambitions. In Cao Cao's poem he wrote: "The old horse resting in a stable aims at a journey of thousands of miles. An ambitious man retains his high aspirations even in old age." Indeed, psychological age is not controlled by time. Mr. Deng Xiaoping was full of vitality when he was 80 years old. During the southern talks, he proposed that "development is the absolute principle" and raised the big sail of China's reform and opening up. Many scientists with grey hairs still maintain exuberant energy and child-like curiosity. In contrast, some youths are emotionally burdened and unable to lift the sails of life. They are exposed to rapid psychological aging. Fortunately, if they change their perceptions and revive their ambitions, they can regain psychological youth.

Exercise is an effective method to maintain a "young" physiological age. I have also noticed that pediatricians generally live a long life. Why? It is because they spend lots of time with children and this benefits their mental health. When Academician Hu Yamei of Beijing Children's

Hospital was nearly 90 years old, her style of speech and her character were still child-like. Academician Hu was proud of her nickname, "Jogging Hu", because she often walked very briskly and seemed young as a result. Research by some experts have proven that if a person has good living habits, their physiological age will be much younger than their natural age.

Can you believe this? She is 85 years old.

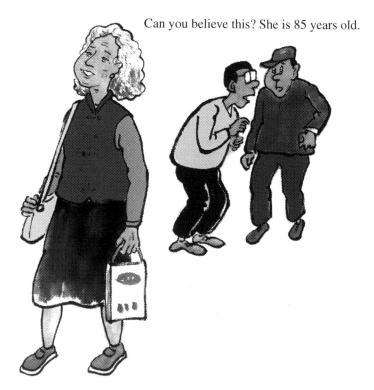

I believe many people have been deeply worried about themselves "getting old before their time." The phenomenon is a result of aging physiologically. Physiological age is a relatively new subject. People often pay more attention to their psychological age while not knowing enough about physiological age or simply consider it as the natural age. In fact, this is not a scientific approach. How can people stay young physiologically? Various experiments have shown that people's beliefs and expectations can affect their bodies. I once read a report on a group of people who were over 70 years old. They were required to participate in activities suitable for young people under 20 years old for some time, that is, they were guided to change their psychological age. As a result, their memory and agility of vision and hearing improved accordingly. On the contrary, a group of middle-aged people in their 40s were asked to shut off from the outside world and resist changes. It turned out that their psychological and physiological reactions were far worse than those of their peers after some time. The experiment shows that our opinions, expectations and mental state greatly affect our bodies. Though physical exercises, muscle development, as well as leisure and rest alone are important aspects, the role of continuous "rejuvenation" in physiological age and psychological age is irreplaceable.

High-income people age fast

Studies have found that high-income people age very quickly. For those aged 30–50, their level of dehydroepiandrosterone, which reflects the physiological function of the body, is only 60% of the average value of normal people of the same age, which means their physiological age is often 10–13 years older than their natural age. A survey conducted by the Chinese Academy of Sciences in 2006 showed that the average life expectancy of intellectuals in China is only 58 years, which is ten years lower than the national average life expectancy, and the phenomenon of early deaths in this class of people is growing. Among people aged 25–59, the female mortality rate is 10.4%, while the male mortality rate is 16.5%. Why is this happening? I believe the "killers" causing people to age fast are the pressures of life, mental stress, and irregularly changing lifestyles.

There was a study on the physiological age and psychological age of different occupational groups. The chosen subjects included 179 industrial workers, 184 teachers and 174 managers of enterprises. The physiological variables closely related to the degree of aging of the chosen subjects and the indicators reflecting the psychological aging were tested. Then, their physiological age and psychological age were calculated. Results showed significant differences in physiological age among industrial workers, teachers and managers of enterprises. Still, there was no evident difference in psychological age (see Table 3). For the case of the actual age being lower than the physiological age, the psychological age, or both, the

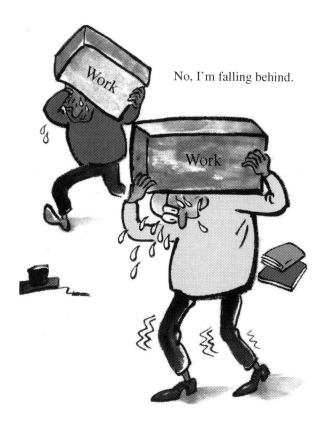

No, I'm falling behind.

Table 3: Physiological age and psychological age of different occupational groups.

Level	Number of people surveyed	Physiological age/year		Psychological age/year	
		$\bar{x} \pm s\bar{x}$	$\bar{x} \pm s\bar{x}^a$	$\bar{x} \pm s\bar{x}$	$\bar{x} \pm s\bar{x}^a$
Industrial workers	179	47.8 ± 6.4	47.61 ± 0.19	49.1 ± 7.0	48.89 ± 0.29
Teachers	184	44.8 ± 9.7	47.12 ± 0.16	45.9 ± 9.4	48.10 ± 0.25
Managers of enterprises	174	48.9 ± 6.0	46.72 ± 0.15	50.7 ± 6.2	48.55 ± 0.23

proportion of industrial workers was significantly higher than that of teachers and managers of enterprises. It shows that manual workers are more likely to "get old before their time" than knowledge workers or those work both manually and mentally.

Table 4: The proportion of people whose physiological age and psychological age are higher than the actual age in all occupational groups.

Group	Total number of people	PhA > CA		PsA > CA		PhA > (PhA + PsA) > CA	
		Number of people	Percentage/%	Number of people	Percentage/%	Number of people	Percentage/%
Industrial workers	179	91	50.84**	122	68.16**	74	41.34**
Teachers	184	51	27.72**	83	45.11	35	19.02
Managers of enterprises	174	22	12.64	77	44.25	13	7.47

Through χ2 test, **P < 0.01; PhA: physiological age; PsA: psychological age; CA: calendar age

The proportion of teachers was also higher than that of managers of enterprises, which indicates that knowledge workers have more chances for "getting old before their time" than those work both manually and mentally (see Table 4).

Middle age is the protection period of life

Chinese author Ba Jin once said, "Beautiful middle age is the mature period in life. For people in this period, life is as broad as the sea and sky, and they are free to go anywhere they want." People often label middle-aged people as "in the prime of life." What age group do middle-aged people actually belong in?

It is commonly believed that people around 40 years old are considered middle-aged. Generally speaking, it is in line with our country's customs to say that people enter middle age at the age of 29 and become "old" at the age of 60. The middle-aged people referred to here are people aged between 29 and 59. From the perspective of growth and development, most people have enter their peak by the age of 25. People start maturing at the age of 30, and the total weight of their brains begins to decrease. At 40–50 years old, people gradually become long-sighted. Their immunity declines and the number of lymphocytes with anti-cancer function drops significantly. Health begins to decline progressively from there.

In 1991, the WHO redivided the life cycle: youth — under 44 years old, middle age — 45–59 years old, early old age — 60–74 years old, older old — 75–89 years old, long-living oldest old — 90 years old and older. In recent years, a study was conducted in the United States to test 20–70-year-old people's ability to solve daily problems. The test results suggest that the order of wisdom periods of life is: 45–49 years old, 30–39 years old, 50–59 years old, 60–69 years old, and 70 years old when there are signs of intelligence decline. In other words, 40–49 years old is the wisest period in life.

Middle age can be said to mark the autumn of life and the time of harvest. It is the wisest period in life. Moreover, the development of tissues and organs is completed and people reach maturity physically and mentally by middle age. By this time, the body's responses to the internal and external environment are fixed, and most people have the physical and mental quality and conditions to cope with heavy and complicated loads. However, in reality, the health condition of middle-aged people is not so optimistic. "Increasing work pressure, heavy burdens of life and great psychological burdens" are three major issues that challenge the health of middle-aged people. Middle-aged people have rich working experience and abundant mental and physical capacity. Most of them are the pillars of their companies, and they undertake complex and weighty tasks at work. Middle-aged people are also the main sources of family income. They carry heavy burdens as they have to support the elderly and raise children. The elderly can rebuke the generation younger than them, and the young can complain about the strictness of their parents. Nevertheless, the middle-aged have nobody to blame and are obliged to take on the hard work of caring for their families and advancing their careers courageously. The physical exhaustion caused by all this increased pressure has become a distinct turning point for the health of middle-aged people. In the 1980s, writer Shen Rong wrote a novel called *At Middle Age* (Ren dao zhongnian), of which the leading character. Dr. Lu Wenting's image caused hot debates in society. At that time, the "four modernizations" were ongoing, and many middle-aged people worked immensely hard while facing various pressures. Many people led a life similar to Dr. Lu's. They worked, suffered, struggled, and made progress. They either made achievements or died wearily... The novel authentically reflected the real life of the middle-aged at that time. Forty years have passed, but the plight of middle-aged people has not changed much.

Middle age is the protection period of life. In the past ten years, there have been severe cases of premature aging and untimely death of middle-aged people in our country, especially amongst middle-aged intellectuals. They are increasingly attracting the attention of the nation. Take Shenzhen as an example. Among all the elites who entered the special economic zone to develop their careers, 3,000 middle-aged intellectuals have died at the average age of 51.2, which is 25.2 years less than the average life expectancy in Guangdong Province in the second national census. According to a survey conducted by the China Institute of Sport Science, the average age of death of intellectuals in Beijing's Innovation hub, Zhongguancun, is 53.34 years old, compared with 58.52 years old a decade ago. Ten years later, the intellectuals in Zhongguancun have advanced their average age of death by 5.18 years. "Ambitions fade when one reaches the middle age." When people reach the age of 35, many of them feel that they are getting old. A bitter taste of helplessness and a sense of detachment from following their fate emerges. They become accustomed to everything in reality. They lose the passion and determination of youth, as they have almost everything they should have and are indifferent to what they do not have.

In fact, middle age is the most precious, wonderful and eventful period in life. Middle-aged people "let ambitions fade" with ease, but "should not revive their ambitions." Middle-aged people have many physiological traits. It is one-sided to generalize them only by "being in the prime of life", which can easily lead to premature aging and premature death. We need to acknowledge that middle-aged people are under great pressure in all aspects and their health is likely to decline. We need to realize that the incidence rate of disease and mortality rate of middle-aged people are higher than those of the elderly. Malignant diseases of the elderly are also mostly caused by hidden hazards from middle age. Given these special circumstances of middle-aged people, we should pay full attention to their healthcare in this period in order to give full play to the talents of middle-aged people and make this prime of life count for them, in order that they may take on the important task of backing the great rejuvenation of China. Middle-aged people should pay adequate attention

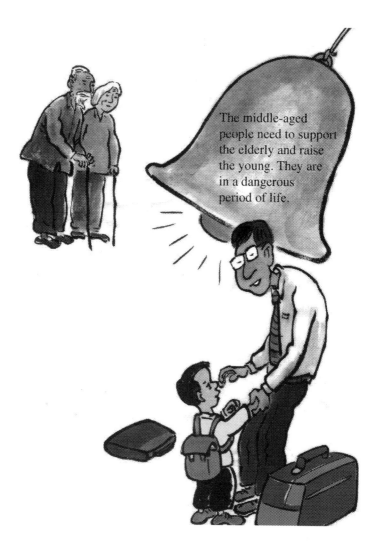

to their physiological changes without being too anxious. Corresponding self-care measures can be taken to build a solid foundation for health, so that they can achieve the purpose of prolonging life. These measures include: reasonable arrangement of work, ensuring sufficient sleep, doing physical exercises, having a healthy diet, and emotional self-control. Investment in health is indispensable for the sake of making greater contributions to the nation, society and family.

Section B

Health is Determined by a Healthy Lifestyle

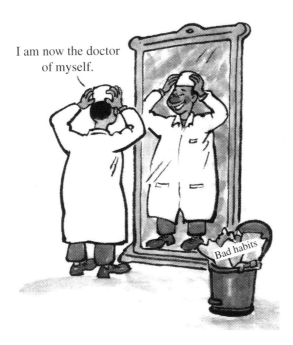

I am now the doctor of myself.

Bad habits

Among factors affecting human health, heredity, social environment, natural environment and many other are beyond our control. Only ours way of life can be chosen and controlled by ourselves. Therefore, we should remember that the best doctor is oneself: my health is in my own hands.

Factors that affect health

There are many factors that affect health, which can be divided into internal and external factors in general. Heredity is the internal factor that accounts for about 15% of all aspects of human health and physical traits. Simply put, heredity is the passing on of biological traits from parents and even grandparents, which will affect the health condition of the second or the third generation. If both parents are short-sighted, their children will mostly be the same. If parents are short in stature, their children will not be tall in general. People's appearance, body shape, diseases and other conditions are mostly related to genes.

On the other hand, external factors are mainly the social environment, natural climate, medical conditions and lifestyle, of which lifestyle has the greatest impact, up to 60%. Thus, heredity is not the most important factor affecting health, lifestyle is. Lifestyle is an amalgamation of living habits and awareness formed by the influence of social culture, economy, customs and family. One of the biggest differences between lifestyle and other factors affecting health is that lifestyle can be chosen by ourselves. We can control it and change it so as to make our life healthier. Choosing a good lifestyle can allow us to maintain our health. In contrast, a bad lifestyle can put us at risk of illnesses: diabetes, peptic ulcer and cardiovascular and cerebrovascular diseases, and greatly increase our risk of getting cancer. The mortality rate of people over 45 years old living unhealthy lifestyle is several times higher than that of people with healthy lifestyles. Therefore, the first step towards health and slowing down aging should be the chioce of a healthy lifestyle.

Lifestyle diseases are the top killer of human health

In the past, the level of human development and knowledge was low, thus, human health was mainly affected by infectious diseases, parasitic diseases, nutritional deficiencies and other diseases. With the development of social productivity and the improvement of living standards, the impact of infectious diseases accompanied by poverty on health has taken a back seat. The diseases caused by unhealthy lifestyle have become the main factors threatening people's health. Data from the WHO shows that with the increase of life expectancy, lifestyle-related conditions appear when the global infant mortality drops below 15 per thousand. Lifestyle diseases refer to physical or psychological diseases caused by people's unhealthy behaviors in all aspects of daily life such as food, clothing, housing, transportation and entertainment, as well as social, economic, spiritual and cultural factors.

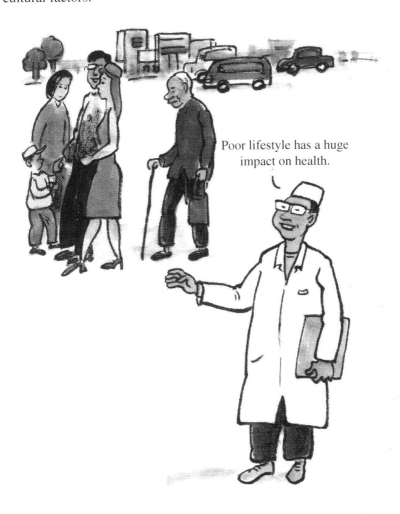

Poor lifestyle has a huge impact on health.

Lifestyle diseases include cardiovascular diseases, stroke, cancer, chronic respiratory diseases and diabetes. These are also called "chronic diseases" by some people because they are mainly chronic and noncommunicable diseases.

Chronic diseases not only appear in developed countries but are also spreading rapidly in developing countries. They have become the "number one killer" endangering people's health. The World Health Statistics 2002 pointed out that death, onset of disease and disability caused by non-communicable diseases accounted for about 60% of all deaths and 47% of the global burden of disease, and were expected to rise to 73% and 60% by 2020, respectively. Therefore, in 2005 the WHO published a report entitled *Preventing Chronic Diseases: A Vital Investment*, pointing out that chronic diseases are the most critical reason for deaths in the world. Deaths caused by chronic diseases account for about 60% of all deaths, and 80% of all deaths from chronic diseases occur in low-income and middle-income countries. It has been predicted that the total deaths caused by infectious diseases, maternal and perinatal diseases and nutritional deficiencies will decline by 3% in the next 10 years, while the number of deaths from chronic diseases caused by lifestyle will increase by 17%. In other words, the threat of lifestyle-related chronic diseases to human beings will become severe. If we still do not take urgent action, an estimated 388 million people will die due to chronic diseases in the next ten years.

Chronic diseases can seriously affect the quality of life of patients and cause premature death, they have huge, negative and underestimated economic impacts on families, communities and the whole society. In China, the results of the "Survey on Nutrition and Health Status of Chinese Residents" jointly released by the Ministry of Health, the Ministry of Science and Technology and the National Bureau of Statistics in 2004 show that, instances of chronic diseases are also steadily increasing and morbidity is on the rise. The number of people, families and communities threatened gradually grows. Apart from major infectious diseases, chronic diseases have become the main health hazard for urban and rural residents in our country. The burden of disease caused by chronic diseases is also getting heavier, accounting for more than 70% of deaths and more than 60% of the total burden of disease. It was estimated that in the ten years between 2006 and 2015, premature death of patients due to heart disease, stroke and diabetes would lead to a loss of gross national income of 558 billion US dollars, making the impacts on the macroeconomy of our country a considerable one. According to the analysis of the top three causes of deaths published in China, the proportion of unhealthy lifestyle to biological factors in cardiovascular diseases is 45.7%: 29.0%, in cerebrovascular diseases it is 43.3%: 36.0%, and in malignant tumors it is 43.6%: 45.9%. These three types of conditions account for 67.6% of all causes of deaths. In other words, two-thirds of people die from illnesses related to unhealthy lifestyles currently.

The main risk factors for chronic diseases are unhealthy diet, insufficient exercise and smoking

The WHO report points out that the risk factors causing chronic diseases are common and variable, and the most important three are unhealthy diet, lack of exercise and smoking. These risk factors are the causes of the majority of deaths of patients of chronic diseases in all regions of the world, of all age groups, and for both men and women.

First of all, bad eating habits are the basic causes of chronic lifestyle diseases. In our country, we have enjoyed increasing material abundance and the rapid development of cultural exchanges between China and the West. As a result, people's diets rich in whole grains and vegetables, with oil, eggs, fish and meat being rationed in the 1950s to 1970s, have changed into the current "three-high" structure — high fat, high protein and high calories. The dietary structure of urban residents, with excessive consumption of livestock meat and fat and inadequate intake of cereals. According to the survey, the average daily fat consumption of urban residents increased from 37 grams in 1992 to 44 grams in 2002, and the proportion of fat intake has reached 36% which exceeds the 30% limit recommended by WHO. Nevertheless, the proportion of cereal intake was only 47%, which was evidently lower than the standard range of 55%–65% recommended by the Chinese Nutrition Society. Fat intake exceeding the standard limit is the main factor causing overnutrition. Overnutrition has led to a significant increase in the number of people suffering from being overweight and obese, which are the mutual risk factors for cardiovascular and cerebrovascular diseases, diabetes, malignant tumors and other chronic diseases. When the body is overweight or obese, adverse metabolic changes will occur in the body, including increased blood pressure, "bad" cholesterol and resistance to insulin. This results in hyperlipidemia, high cholesterol and decreased glucose tolerance. By this time, the body is already at high risk of the onset of disease. If people don't pay attention to their unhealthy living habits, they may very well end up as patients of chronic diseases: high blood pressure, coronary disease, diabetes, etc. If people still do not adopt a healthy lifestyle to intervene the diseases, it will eventually lead to damage to the heart, brain and renal function, disability and even death.

Apart from the influence of dietary factors, lack of exercise is the second largest risk factor for chronic diseases. After all, it is because our living environment has changed dramatically. Unlike in the past, most of us today take the elevator instead of stairs, commute by car, do housework with electrical appliances, work with computers, walk less, and have fewer physical activities.

Every year, many students join our institute. But the main players of basketball and table tennis at the sports grounds are still the same old faces. Even if young people have joined, it is difficult for them to become the main players mainly because they do not seem to like sports. As long as I have time, I will try my best to arrange activities like swimming and playing ball games. I see that many young men and women go to restaurants, watch movies, play poker and play games online after work. However, there are not many people changing into sportswear and exercising.

I once discussed this topic with several young people, who complained and said, "Doing exercises every day? Uh, we are too busy working and we are not professional athletes!" Well, I am also an ordinary person. My work is also hectic. Why is it the case that I can still keep exercising? The key is to attach importance to and develop the habit of exercising. The fundamental reasons for the appearance of more and more "heavyweights (pangdun)" in modern society are insufficient exercise and imbalanced diets. The term heavyweight (pangdun) is popular, and it actually means overweight or obese, a condition mainly caused by the abnormality of excessive fat accumulated in the body.

Body mass index (BMI) is the most useful standard for the measurement of abnormal bodyweight and obesity. It is defined as a person's weight in kilograms divided by the square (kg/m^2) of height in meters. A BMI that equals to or surpasses 25 indicates that one is "overweight" and a BMI that equals to or exceeds 30 means one is "obese". I would like to tell you some alarming figures. WHO's recent forecast shows that about 1.6 billion adults (over 15 years old) worldwide are overweight and at least 400 million adults are obese. Every year, 2.6 million people worldwide die of health issues due to being overweight or obese. More than 2 million people die of lack of physical activity, and 65%–85% of adults in each country suffer from damaged health due to lack of sufficient physical activity. Overweight and obesity were once regarded as problems that only exist in high-income countries, but it is a rising trend in low-income countries and middle-income countries, especially in cities. Data from China's Ministry of Health in 2002 showed that about 200 million adults in our nation are overweight and more than 60 million are obese. The overweight rate has reached 22.8% and the obesity rate is 7.1%. Compared with 1992, the overweight rate and obesity rate of Chinese residents have increased by 38.6% and 80.6%, respectively. And, the rate of adults over 18 years old being overweight and obese have increased by 40.7% and 97.2%, respectively. The cumulative number of people who are overweight and obese has increased by nearly 100 million. Growth trends like these are really worrying.

Finally, there is the problem of smoking. It is an indisputable fact that smoking can increase the risk of various chronic diseases. Tobacco contains dozens of toxic substances. Many studies in epidemiology have confirmed that smoking can lead to the onset and development of chronic diseases such as coronary disease, lung cancer, chronic bronchitis and chronic obstructive pulmonary disease. At present, there are about 350 million smokers in China, and more than half of the non-smokers are also harmed by "second-hand smoke." According to a 2006 survey published by *The Lancet*, an authoritative international medical journal, which collected data from 52 countries' national health surveys, at least 4.8 million people worldwide die of smoking every year. WHO predicts that if the current smoking pattern continues, the number of deaths in each year will double to 10 million by 2020.

The three unhealthy lifestyle components, unhealthy diet, insufficient exercise and smoking, and the related spreading chronic disease, are becoming

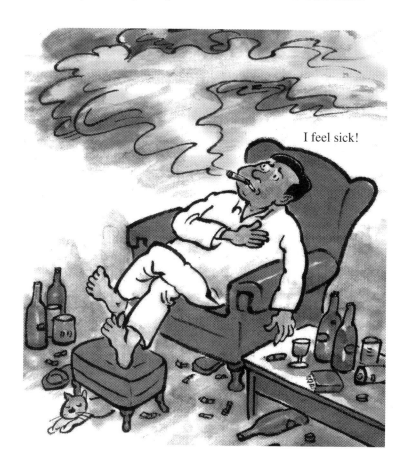

I feel sick!

more and more common in developing countries. High blood pressure is especially worth mentioning. Its prevalence rate in China has been continuously rising for the past 50 years. According to the three national high blood pressure sampling surveys in 1958–1959, 1979–1980 and 1991, as well as the health status survey of Chinese residents in 2002, the prevalence rate of high blood pressure among people over 15 years old is 5.1%, 7.7%, 13.6% and 17.6%, respectively, indicating a massive upward trend. It is estimated that there are 160 million people with high blood pressure with an increase of more than 3 million each year. What is even more worrying is that less than 1/3 of patients know that they are ill, and only about 1/4 of patients are receiving treatment. The control rate of blood pressure is only 6.1%, that is to say, the blood pressure of most patients with high blood pressure has not been effectively controlled.

In addition, patients with coronary disease increase by 1.1 million every year in China. The number of people who get myocardial infarction every year is half a million, and the number of existing patients is 2 million. There are 2 million new cases of stroke every year, and there are 6–7 million existing patients currently. There is a new case of stroke every 15 seconds, and one person dies of stroke every 21 seconds. Nearly 3 million people die of cardiovascular and cerebrovascular diseases every year, with roughly, 1.5 million dying of each disease, respectively. Among the surviving patients, about 3/4 of them have lost their ability to work to varying degrees, and the treatment costs even more if they are severely disabled. The annual medical cost for cardiovascular and cerebrovascular diseases amounts to 110 billion yuan, translating to a heavy economic burden to patients and society.

What's more, nearly 2 million new cases of tumors are added every year in our country, and about 1.5 million people die of cancer. In 2005, medical expenses of cancer accounted for about 10% of the country's total health expenses, exceeding 90 billion yuan.

......

What a grim situation this is!

My health is in my own hands

As I have emphasized, health is closely related to lifestyle. A healthy lifestyle can improve people's health and prevent diseases, while unhealthy living habits and behaviors will endanger one's health and bring diseases to people. The kind of lifestyle we choose depends on ourselves. Without exception, we bear the consequences of our choices.

I used to enjoy hamburgers and meat very much. But ever since my experience of a heart attack, I have paid great attention to my diet and adjusted my diet accordingly. Now, I generally don't eat fat meat anymore. I eat a vegetable salad at the beginning of a meal and urge myself to eat more vegetables at every meal.

Studies show that the lifestyle of 20 years can determine one's physical condition at the end of the 20 years. Many common and fatal diseases are invisible and hard to notice at the beginning, and it often takes 10 or 15 years before symptoms develop. Although the consequences of disability and lethality mainly occur in middle age and when one becomes more elderly, the onset of the disease occurs in the adolescent period. Many young people have boudless energy, thus they pay attention to making money or playing rather than caring for their health and restricting their lifestyle. Originally, many health experts advocate a "full breakfast, good lunch and small dinner." However, in reality, many white-collar workers and working people choose "no breakfast, passable lunch and full dinner." The consequences caused by such eating habits are very severe. People can get cholecystitis (gallbladder inflamation) if they don't eat breakfast for a long time. Stomach troubles will happen if people don't eat lunch on time. If people overeat at night,

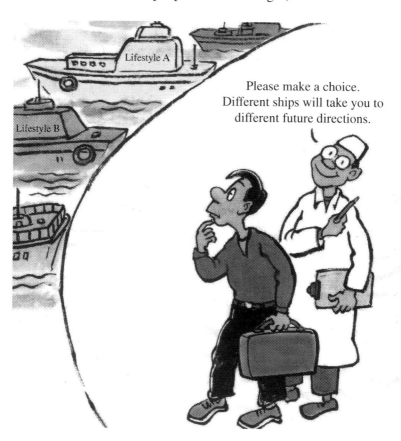

their intestines and stomach will have to work overtime instead of taking a rest, which is very harmful to the body; it is pure common sense! Add to this, smoking, drinking, going to bed late and getting up late, and not exercising ...Unhealthy lifestyles have been developed unconsciously, and potential crises unknown to people are quietly approaching.

In recent years, the patients of chronic diseases, which originally have been older people, are getting younger. We now know that almost 50% of deaths from chronic diseases occur prematurely among people under 70 years old. In low-income countries and middle-income countries, middle-aged people are particularly vulnerable to chronic diseases. Compared with high-income countries, people in these countries are younger when they have the onset of illness. They suffer from diseases for a longer period of time, and are often accompanied by preventable complications. Futhermore, they age faster.

Chronic diseases are preventable and treatable

Chronic diseases are different from infectious diseases and cannot be prevented with vaccines and drugs. Many people think that it is useless to treat diseases that are "chronic", so they give up active treatment. This is a wrong attitude. The main causes of chronic diseases are known and mostly caused by unhealthy personal behaviors. If these risk factors are eliminated, at least 80% of heart disease, stroke, type II diabetes and chronic obstructive pulmonary disease, and more than 40% of cancer cases can be avoided.

Human beings have mastered the means to prevent and treat chronic diseases, meaning that we can altogether avoid the heavy burden of disability caused by chronic diseases. American scholars have predicted that it will cost 10 billion US dollars to increase the average life expectancy of American adults by one year. However, if people exercise regularly, do not smoke, drink less and eat properly, they can increase their average life expectancy by 11 years with little cost. A "Ninth Five-Year Plan" key research in China indicates that there are very few patients with severe high blood pressure, and 85% of patients are below the medium level. For patients with low-level and medium-level high blood pressure, they can relieve their diseases to a certain extent through the improvement of lifestyles such as dietary adjustment, exercise and rest, which can effectively reduce the incidence rate of coronary disease and stroke. In this way, the cost of disease prevention investment is minimized and the effect is maximized. Some studies have shown that every yuan spent on comprehensive prevention and treatment of patients with high blood pressure in communities can save 8.59 yuan for cardiovascular and cerebrovascular treatment. What is more important is that patients suffer less and their families are relieved. Medical expenses are saved and the whole society benefits.

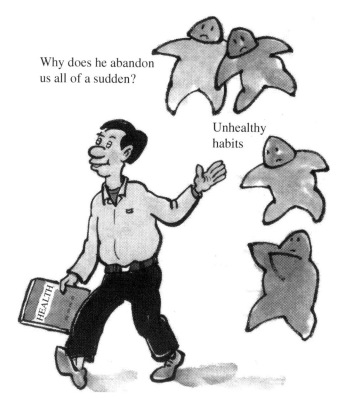

Why does he abandon us all of a sudden?

Unhealthy habits

Dr. Leicester from the Department of Public Health, University of California, USA, conducted a 9-year follow-up survey of about 7,000 males and females aged 11 to 75 from different socio-economic classes and with different lifestyles. The results have proved that people's daily lifestyle is closely related to their health. He summed up a set of concise and healthy lifestyle habits.

1. Exercise regularly (the amount of exercise should be suitable for one's physical condition).
2. Have seven or eight hours of sleep every day.
3. Have breakfast regularly.
4. Have more frequent, but smaller, meals (4–5 meals a day).
5. Do not smoke.
6. Do not drink or only drink a small amount of low-alcohol wine.
7. Control one's body weight (not less than 10% and not more than 20% of standard body weight).

My friend, how is your lifestyle? When we hold the remote control in our hands and turn on electrical appliances using our devices or voices instead of our arms, do we realize that our muscles are shrinking and the function of our limbs is deteriorating? Therefore, we should not only "watch what we eat" but also "move our legs" and increase physical activity.

Section C

The Five Cornerstones of Health

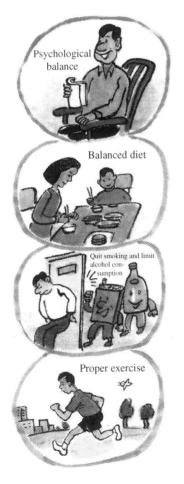

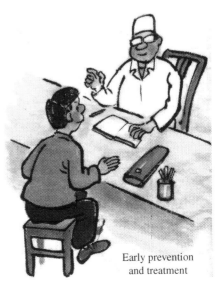

Life is limited and health is priceless. Health is a one-way street: returning to a good health from a poor condition is difficult. We should take care of our own health and improve the awareness of self-care. Having a natural age of 84 years, a physiological age of 40 years, and psychological of 30 years is by no means impossible.

Among the factors affecting human health, genetic factors and environmental factors account for only 15% and 17%, medical conditions account for 8%, and one's attitude toward life and lifestyle accounts for 60%. The ratio shows that the most important factor influencing human health and longevity is personal choice. In other words, everyone's mental health, lifestyle behaviors and habits are the key factors that determine health and longevity. The state of a person's health is largely the result of his/her choice of lifestyle. Professor Hong Zhaoguang has mentioned before that health has four cornerstones: psychological balance, reasonable diet, smoking and limiting alcohol consumption, and proper exercise. I agree with them very much and have one more cornerstone to add: early prevention and treatment.

Psychological balance

Of all the adverse factors, the ones that can make people die prematurely are negative mood and passive mentalities such as worry, fear, greed, cowardice, jealousy and hatred.

—— Hu Tianlande

Psychological balance is the most critical in all of the cornerstones of health. I believe that the essential essence of the regimen is mental balance, which is vital yet hard to achieve. A person with a positive attitude is perceived as a young person, while a negative mentality is most likely to make people age. Zheng Xiaoyu, former director of the National Medical Products Administration, turned white-haired within the few months after he was investigated and sentenced to death of corruption. The main reason for that is the large psychological setback.

A healthy mentality means that when we encounter difficulties, setbacks and sudden changes in our life, we can still achieve psychological harmony, mental stability, and can adequately manage the situations and rule out unfavorable influences. Nevertheless, in real life, people are often bothered by negative emotions such as worry, fear, greed, cowardice, jealousy and hatred.

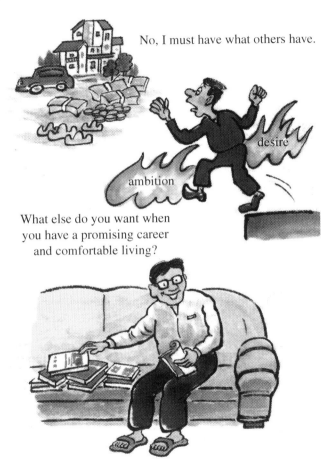

These negative emotions can result in the decline of human immune function, sub-health, and even various diseases. Scientific research shows that the anti-cancer function of human body will decline by more than 20% when one's mood is low. As the ancients said, "a healthy spirit lies within a healthy body."

As far as I can remember, at the beginning of the spread of SARS in 2003, many people fell into panic and believed in rumors because they did not know enough about this disease. In some places, many people frantically bought salt, vinegar, Radix Isatidis (a herbal medicine) and other items. In other areas, people even tried to block roads to cut off the connection with the outside. All of these look ridiculous now. At that time, they were mainly psychological issues. I had a patient who had been infected with SARS. She was a primary school teacher. She continued wearing masks every time she came back for return visits even after she was cured and SARS had been eradicated for months. I talked to her and it turned out that she was afraid of infecting her colleagues and family members, so she did not dare to take off the masks and she shut herself away from others. I told her that there was no need to worry at all. She could work and live normally without infecting others.

A depressed mood is a health killer

Medical research shows that mood is closely related to human health. When a person encounters mental pressure and is in a bad psychological state, experiencing tension, anger and anxiety, abnormal physiological changes can result. If this occurs repeatedly for a long time, it may gradually evolve from functional changes to organic damages.

Psychologists have conducted an experiment to study the relationship between emotion and health. They locked two monkeys in a cage. One was free to move and the other was tied to the edge of the cage and could not move freely. There was an insulation rod on one side of the cage. When the experimenter electrified the cage every half minute, the free monkey was free to seize the insulating rod to avoid electric shock. After the experiment began, the free monkey was on tenterhooks, always thinking about grabbing the insulating rod every half a minute to avoid being shocked. By contrast, the tied-up monkey could not escape, so it resigned itself to the shocks and stayed calm. After a period of time, the physical examination of the two monkeys revealed that the free monkey had an ulcer disease, while the tied-up monkey stayed healthy. The experiment shows that long-term stress can be the cause of diseases.

It is not uncommon to encounter diseases or even accidents induced by excessive emotional excitement in daily life. I recall that on the night of October 18, 1981, the Chinese men's soccer team defeated Kuwait, the leader of Asian soccer back then, 3–0 in the World Cup qualifying match. A spectator died in the stands due to a heart attack after the match. In November of the same year, the Chinese and Japanese women's volleyball teams competed for the World Cup. After the match, nine spectators with heart diseases had worsened conditions, and two of them died despite medical attention. The reason for their relapses was that they were too excited.

Researchers have found through investigation that people who are stubborn, argumentative, impatient, angry and grumpy are most likely to get coronary diseases. Experts investigated more than 1,000 stroke patients and found that 75% of cases were induced by psychological factors. Patients with heart diseases or high blood pressure, particularly, should not get too excited. Other diseases such as cancer, diabetes and ulcers are also closely related to emotions.

Depressed people are prone to tumor

German scholar Dr. Balterus investigated more than 8,000 cancer patients and found that the onset of cancer of most patients occurred under severe mental stress like disappointment, loneliness and chagrin. Dr. Steven Greer observed 160 patients with breast tumors admitted to London hospitals. Some of the patients suffered from cancer, and some did not. He found that 60% of non-cancer patients could express their emotions freely, while only 1/3 of breast cancer patients could do the same. The remaining 2/3 tended to suppress their emotions. In the 1980s, 200 gastric cancer patients were surveyed in Shanghai and it was found that they shared the characteristics of long-term emotional depression and disharmonious families. Data from a group of randomized and controlled surveys in Beijing revealed that 76% of cancer patients had experienced adverse psychological stimulation in their lives, while only 32% of non-cancer patients had experienced evident adverse psychological stimulation. These facts show that long-term mental stress, emotional suppression, depression, pessimism and disappointment are harmful mental states and are strong cancer promoters.

Therefore, I personally think that among all five cornerstones of health, the first one, psychological balance, is most important. Longevity villages have become popular in recent years. The people in those villages may not have the same eating habits or do similar exercises, but one thing they have in common is psychological balance. Psychological balance is nevertheless a great challenge for many, especially young and middle-aged working adults who form the backbone of companies/organizations. Hu Tianlande, a famous medical philosopher, has a famous saying: "Of all the adverse factors, the ones that can make people die prematurely are negative mood and passive mentalities such as worry, fear, greed, cowardice, jealousy and hatred." Let me take the onset of tumor as an example. Usually, there are two genes related to the onset of tumor in the human body at the same time, which are tumor suppressor genes and oncogenes, respectively. It may not be common knowledge that, in fact, human oncogenes produce more than 3,000 cancer cells everyday. However, why doesn't everyone get cancer? This is because there are 9 billion lymphocytes in leukocytes of human blood, of which 5%–10% are natural killer cells (NK cells). The NK cells have the most potent toxic effect on human tumor cells. Their duty is to attack and destroy cancer cells. Once natural killer cells spot cancer cells, they will combine with them. In less than five minutes, the substances in natural killer cells will destroy cancer cells and kill them. Generally speaking, it takes 5–10 natural killer cells to eradicate a cancer cell. This is why most people do not have cancer even though the human body produces cancer cells everyday. Cancer cells are killed as soon as they appear. However, psychoneuroimmunology studies have found that the fighting capacity of anti-cancer warriors is closely related to emotions. Negative emotions will weaken their fighting capacity, while positive emotions such as optimism and self-confidence can stimulate their vitality. When one is in a bad mood and feels depressed everyday, the function of the secretory system of natural killer cells will be inhibited. According to test results, the cellular activity of natural killer cells can be reduced by more than 20% when one feels depressed, thus reducing their killing effectiveness and their ability to resist cancer cells. In other words, people who are lonely, worried and often in a bad mood are more likely to get cancer. Therefore, maintaining psychological balance is essential for health and longevity.

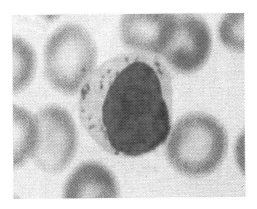

NK cells under light microscope.

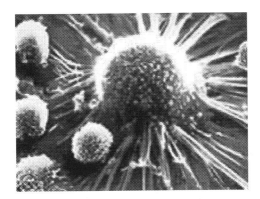

Electron microscope shows that many NK cells are moving toward cancer cells and aggregating.

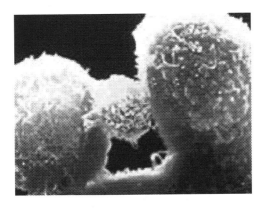

An NK cell attacks cancer cells: cancer cells are on both sides and the NK cell is in the middle.

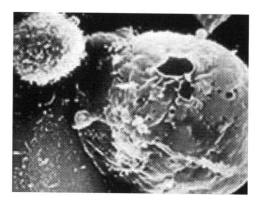

An NK cell penetrates a cancer cell and has left a hole. The cancer cell will die in a very short time.

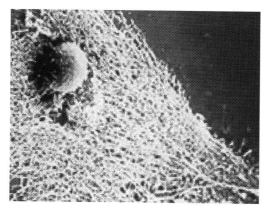

Cancer cells are dead and become fibrosis, and the NK cell can still recover to its original state and continue to search for enemies.

Mental health comes first in self-care and is the key to longevity

One of the important conclusions from the research of many major diseases in the past is that positive and optimistic emotions play an unexpected role in preventing and treating diseases. Taking cancer research as an example: clinical practice shows that positive and optimistic emotions can make malignant tumors change towards a benign state and even have the possibility of diminishing them.

A report published in the German magazine *Science Today* said that researchers surveyed 10,000 men with this question: "Do you think your wife loves you?" The results indicated that the prevalence rate of angina pectoris in men who thought their wives loved them was significantly lower than that the rest of research subjects. Researchers also conducted another experiment. They injected more than 400 people with a type of cold virus. The results showed that among the subjects who had close relationships with three or fewer people, 62% caught a cold. At the same time, only 35% of the subjects who had close relationships with six or more people were sick. Researchers concluded that long-term and harmonious relationships with friends, neighbors and colleagues is a very important immune factor.

People usually think that blind optimism should be avoided when looking at things or making a decision, but optimism is necessary for maintaining physical health. It can be unrealistic optimism sometimes, but

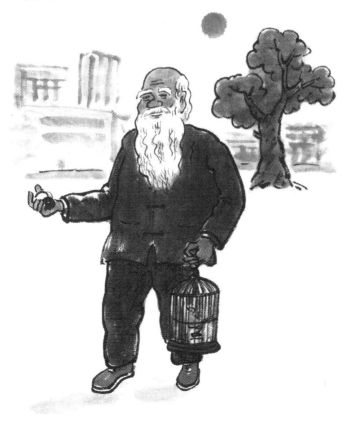

even fantasy is worth recommending. Studies of German scientists have shown that those who are overly practical and realistic are at great risk of depression. A German study of some men suffering from AIDS has shown that the life expectancy of optimistic patients is on average nine months longer than that of patients who worry about death all day long. Optimistic patients said that they fantasized about the possibility of recovery everyday. Through this survey, scientists found that the onset time of AIDS was delayed for optimistic patients who were less realistic.

In short, excessive tension, worry and other negative emotions will lead to dysfunction of the immune system and increase the possibility of illness. On the other hand, by effectively improving the body's immunity, positive and optimistic emotions can not only reduce the probability of illness but also play a positive role in promoting recovery after illness. Therefore, everyone who is "fighting" for the sake of career, especially young and middle-aged elites, must learn to maintain psychological balance.

So, how can we maintain psychological balance?

Persistent Pursuit — The cornerstone of psychological balance

Most people know from experience that in order to achieve psychological balance, one must first have a goal. "If one has a goal to pursue and everything he/she does is to achieve this goal, then unpleasant things around him/her will be ignored." For example, there are many Tibetan Buddhists who overcome unimaginable difficulties such as obstacles of economy, environment and transportation, to "crawl" and kowtow from their hometowns to the Potala Palace to worship their god. It is their firm and devout belief that enables such behavior. Another example is shooting. If you concentrate on hitting the bull's-eye, you won't care for anything else.

As Wang Guowei said in *Notes and Comments on Ci Poetry*, there are three realms of people who have great accomplishments from the past to present. The first realm is "Last night the western breeze, blew withered leaves off trees. I mount the tower high".

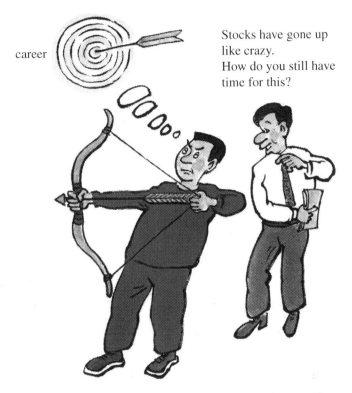

The second realm is "I find my gown too large, but I will not regret; It's worthwhile growing languid for my dear coquette." The third realm is "But in the crowd once and again, I look for her in vain. When all at once I turn my head, I find her there where lantern light is dimly shed." I admire his three realms a lot. They have reflected people's persistent pursuit.

Confucius once said, "They who know the truth are not equal to those who love it, and they who love it are not equal to those who delight in it." It is a beautiful expression for persistent pursuit that also applies to work: for the same job, people with strong professional ability are not as good as those who like the job, and people who like the job are not as good as those who continue in it. In other words, you may not necessarily be very successful even if your professional ability is great. On the contrary, the person who persists in the job can succeed.

Japanese scientists once conducted a 7-year follow-up survey among a group of people aged 40–90. In this group, 60% of them had clear life goals and were designated as Group A; 5% did not have clear life goals and were classified as Group B. The rest 35% had certain life goals but were not clear, and they were classified as Group C. As a result, after seven years, 3,000 people in group B had died of illness or committed suicide, which was double the number of group A, and the cardiovascular and cerebrovascular morbidity in group B was much higher than the other groups. This study tells us that people living in society must have life goals and pursue them.

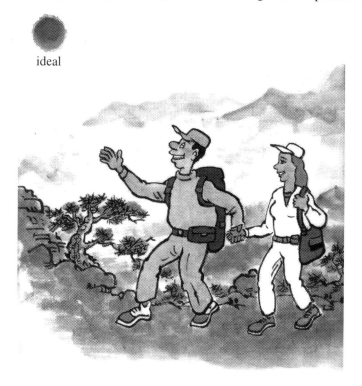

ideal

Pursue persistently, but not blindly

Persistent pursuit is the basis for maintaining psychological balance, but can psychological balance be obtained by blind pursuit? Not necessarily. A person can feel relaxed and happy if he/she has a goal set within reachable range to pursue but is not harsh on him/herself, and at the same time knows how to appreciate his/her achievements. If the goal is set too high and completely beyond the scope of one's ability, just like climbing a ladder to pick the moon, stepping on a box to lift the box or other foolish things, good mental health cannot be maintained.

"Information Technology" in English is abbrievated as IT. Due to fierce competition and high tension, many people interpret the abbreviation of the profession as "I'm tired." In the IT industry, people are considered old when they reach the age of 40, because the industry is developing rapidly and the elimination rate is very high. People usually can't keep up with the pace when they reach their 40s. Excessive pursuit often leads to psychological imbalance.

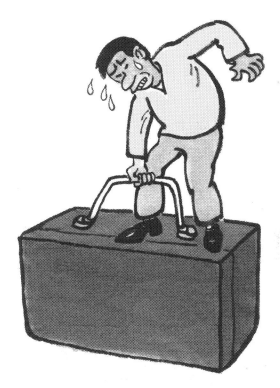

Be kind to yourself, be kind to frustrations

In the process of pursuing goals, we should expect setbacks. That is to say, we should have a strong "resilience quotient" in order to have a balanced mind. Compared with IQ and EQ, "resilience quotient" is sometimes more important, especially for people at work. As we all know, one cannot always be successful and will encounter setbacks of one kind or another. How should we deal with setbacks? I often think of Lao Zi's words: "Good luck and bad luck are foundations of each other."

As a story goes, a wife was always nagging her husband for not being motivated to excel. Later, her husband worked hand and was finally promoted. He became a people magnet and enjoyed the finer things in life that money could buy. Eventually, however, the husband divorced his wife for another women. Sometimes, people's sincere expectations can have opposite results. We should adjust our mindsets, embrace pressure with a positive and optimistic attitude, and look for the positive in failures and setbacks, so as to achieve a new psychological balance.

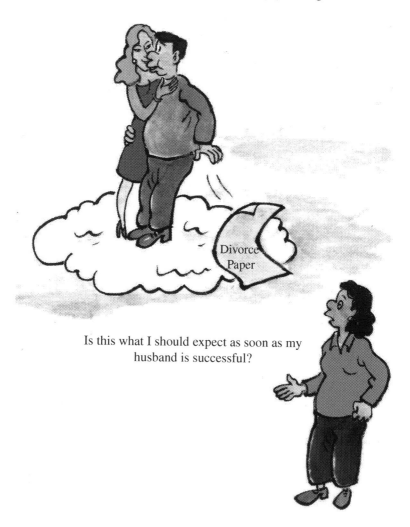

Is this what I should expect as soon as my
husband is successful?

People naturally need respect from others

People who have good relations with others feel good because human beings are social creatures. Where do good relations come from? The biggest difference between human beings and animals is that all of us are born with the need for appreciation and respect. No matter how many shortcomings a person has, you can always find strengths to compliment them on. It is an irrefutable truth that when you know how to appreciate others, you will also gain good relations with them. In 1979, I went to London as an international student. I gained a deep understanding of this when I was studying there. In Britain, our qualifications as Chinese doctors were not recognized. We couldn't go to the wards in hospitals and could only stay in laboratories. At that time, I was eager to broaden my horizons, so I wanted to be able to do both. Hence, I sought permission from one of mentors, Professor Robson, head of the internal medicine department, but my multiple applications were rejected. Later, his secretary saw that I was so persistent and helped me negotiate with the professor. The professor finally agreed to give me 10 minutes to meet him. Ten minutes was too short for me to state my purpose. At that moment, I suddenly remembered that I had read his new book *A Companion to Medical Studies* in the library, so this book became the topic and I talked about its characteristics which I found to be interesting and useful. It linked up the narration of human anatomy, physiology, pathology and diseases, helping students to understand diseases from basic to clinical, with very distinct holistic features.

I readily offered my opinions to show that I understood the meaning of the book. I thought I had left a positive impression on him. He was very happy and talked to me about the process of writing the book. Finally, he agreed to all my requests to visit the wards and other laboratories. To my surprise, he also gave me a new copy of his book which was worth 110 pounds. The conversation between us lasted more than 70 minutes. I received profound inspiration from this experience, sincerely praising the strong points of others, instead of complimenting them with shallow praise, will certainly win their recognition. Forty-one years have passed, and I still have this book on the bookcase directly in front of me. I often look up at the book and remind myself of the virtue of showing appreciation and respect.

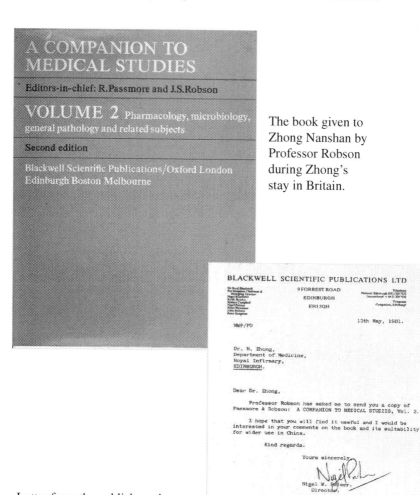

The book given to
Zhong Nanshan by
Professor Robson
during Zhong's
stay in Britain.

Letter from the publisher who
was asked by Professor Robson to
send a book to Zhong Nanshan.

Make use of the team and be good at cultivating yourself

In the process of fighting SARS, we did our work and achieved excellent results of high recovery rate and low mortality rate. One thing that mattered was that we had an excellent team. I knew our team very well. Our team had received better training and had a solid foundation of experience. Therefore, I had confidence and took the initiative to request the Guangdong Province Health Department to send critically ill SARS patients to our institute for centralized treatment. Our team rose to the challenge and sucessfully treated many of these cases.

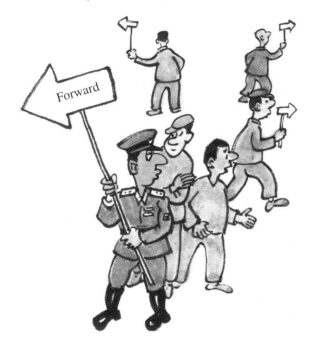

The cultivation of a team is essential. To form an excellent team, we need to discover the strengths and weaknesses of team members and complement one another, rather than put each other down. Additionally, we should be tolerant and fair to people as no one can stand injustice. It is normal to have differences and contradictions in any team, but as a team leader, one should not only pursue peace of mind among team members but also unite the team so it can perform its work. We should strive to train our professional workers into excellent leaders to share the load. Instead of becoming workaholics, they can become commanders who know how to dispatch troops, who continuously improve themselves and obtain psychological pleasure in self-actualization.

What is the difference between professional workers and excellent leaders? My personal opinion is that their mindsets are different. Professional workers think that they need to surpass others in skills to become paddlers. Whilst excellent leaders may not be able to become paddlers, but they are steersmen who are good at motivating people and creating enthusiasm for work. The professional workers understand technical management, and they know how to get things done. Meanwhile, the excellent leaders understand administrative management and know why to get those things done. In a word, I think we should try not to be workaholics regardless of whether we are professional workers or excellent leaders.

Helping others makes one feel at ease

Scientific research has found that the secretion of biotin in the human body can make people happy, which is what Confucius often said, "benevolent people can live a long life." When you help others solve difficulties, and when your existence brings happiness to the community, you will feel happy and content. In 2007, Hu Hanwei, a 101-year-old man from Zhongshan City, Guangdong Province, climbed the 9,999 steps in Baishui Village, Zengcheng City. He revealed his secret of longevity and said that

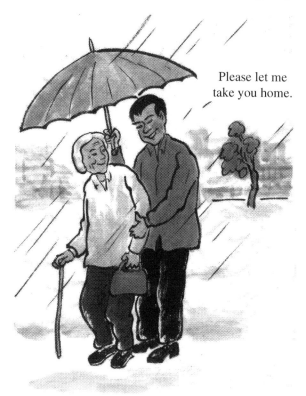

Please let me
take you home.

it was nothing more than doing good deeds. Confucius advocated that "one should first establish one's character in keeping good health", that is, one should first establish a good character. Helping others and being tolerant of others can lead to health and happiness, which has been proven medically. As we all know, monks, nuns and other religious people often live long lives. Their lives are simple, but they have religious beliefs that sustain them.

They think about ways to help the poor everyday. Myraid literature sources show that this mentality can make people happy.

Don't take your work home

It is inevitable to encounter all kinds of problems and setbacks at work, and it is easy to bring the sense of annoyance home from work without noticing. We should take the initiative to manage our emotions, pay attention to our life after work, and avoid bringing home the pressure of work. Family and home should be a haven, a place that makes people feel warm and cozy. If you bring back your negative emotions from work and yell at your family for no reason apparent to them, it will do no good except to cause disputes and intensify conflicts.

After returning home, you should make time for fun, set aside space for rest and recuperation, and spend time with your family. Talk, read, meditate, listen to music, deal with housework, perhaps even do some physical labor, etc., which are all excellent ways to obtain inner peace.

Enjoy life

What kind of person is the happiest? It is critical to know that those who can enjoy themselves are the happiest. Britain's *The Sun* newspaper once held a prize-winning contest on the topic of "What kind of people are the happiest." Among the more than 80,000 letters, the public selected four best answers:

1. An artist who has just finished his work and whistles while admiring it.
2. Children who are building castles out of sand.
3. A mother who is giving her baby a bath.
4. The surgeon who finally saved the life of a critical patient after painstaking operations.

It is not hard to see that these joys are all the joys of process or success from the heart.

The *Health Times* published an article about a retired old man who enjoyed himself and became more and more energetic as he aged. The old man retired for three years, and his symptoms of moderate fatty liver disappeared, blood lipid level became standard, and his weight loss was near 15 kg. He didn't spend money on healthcare products or take any specific drugs. The key was that he had a positive mindset and enjoyed himself in life. People's mood are heavily associated with their physical conditions. Everyone has times of disappointment and helplessness, but what's the use of sighing all day? If you have the ability to solve the problems, try your best to solve them. But if you are unable to do so, you must learn to be content with the situation, in other words, change your mindset.

From my own experience, there are a few things to do in order to be happy. First, we must work. Having work to do will make people happy. Second, we must be full of imagination, be full of hope for the future, always maintain child-like innocence, and know how to enjoy ourselves. Third, we must have love in our hearts, selfless and unconditional love. Fourth, we must have the ability and the skills to help others.

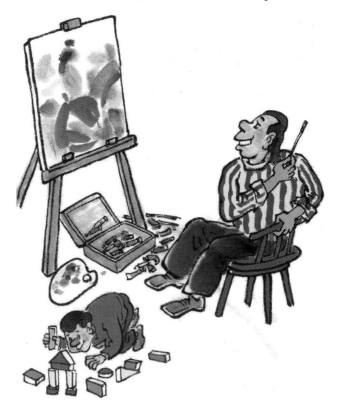

Therefore, I think we should keep in mind these "three joys" with respect to persistent pursuit, helping others, being content and enjoying ourselves. If you can achieve all of these, you can feel good everyday and your work and relationship with the people around you will definitely get better and better.

Find a comfort object — The mysterious power of pets

Some people say that modern society is becoming more and more like a "concrete forest", in which the space for living and activities is becoming smaller, and meaningful communication and interaction between people are becoming less. People are lonelier than before. Under this circumstance, pets such as dogs and cats can be good life partners for people and a kind of comfort object to help people relieve the loneliness of life and regulate their mental health. A study has found that people who own pets go to the hospital less each year than people who do not have pets by 15%–20%.

A 1995 report in the *Journal of the American Heart Association* stated that people who own pet dogs have a lower risk of dying of a heart attack. In 1999, the *Journal of the American Geriatrics Society* reported that pet owners could complete daily activities more quickly, i.e. bathing, dressing, cooking and walking. In 2001, *High Blood Pressure* magazine claimed that when under mental stress, the rise of blood pressure of pet owners is lower. In 2005, the *British Medical Journal* said that keeping pets is of great benefit to the physical and mental health of the elderly and can reduce the risk of the onset of cardiovascular diseases.

I hope to have cats to call my own soon…

Some elderly people are called empty nesters, which means their children or descendants do not live with them. In families like these, the offspring usually go home once a week, and the elderly spend most of their time alone. Therefore, the elders are likely to feel lonely and empty or may even feel abandoned and neglected by others. I suggest that they should keep a pet as an emotional comfort, which is a good way to relieve loneliness.

Professor Zheng Richang and Dr. Fu Na from the Faculty of Psychology of Beijing Normal University found that empty nesters with pets are healthier and more satisfied with their lives than those without pets. Companion animals have provided aspect of cherished non-human social support, such as safety, the feeling of being cherished, being loved and liked, and personal values, etc., they satisfy people's desire for communication and attention, and reduce the negative impact of life pressure and loneliness on people.

The latest research also shows that pets can strengthen people's social communications and enhance relationships between people, thus improving their physical and mental health. There were two people in an experiment, in which one person took a dog out and the other went around alone. They wore different clothings and also exchanged roles, interacting with people from all walks of life. Results showed that the one with the dog interacted with people more frequently no matter how he was dressed. Why do pets make it simple for people to communicate with each other?

This is because pets are a good topic to start a conversation, thus increasing opportunities for pleasant and harmonious social interaction. In this way, it is easy to build friendships. This may be one of the reasons that pet owners are healthier than other people.

Pets help people live longer

A research in Britain showed that after spending several months with a puppy or a kitten, many people felt that the symptoms of some of their recurring diseases had been relieved, including headaches and back pain, etc. In 1992, Australian scientists reported that the blood cholesterol level of people with pets is lower than that of people with similar lifestyles, but no small animals as companions, and so is their heart disease morbidity.

Eric Friedman, a professor at New York University, has found that loving pets help people live a long life. Friedman studied 92 male patients who were recovering from heart diseases and asked them in detail about their lifestyles, including whether they had pets. A year later, 14 out of 92 patients were dead. When looking for the difference between survivors and the deceased, researchers found that people who live alone are more likely to relapse. In contrast, people who keep small animals are more likely to recover. Friedman initially speculated that it was easy for people with puppies to recover because they might have exercised by walking their dogs everyday. However, he also found that people who had raised other animals that did not need walking also recovered better. He then investigated whether the owners of pets were in better health, but it was

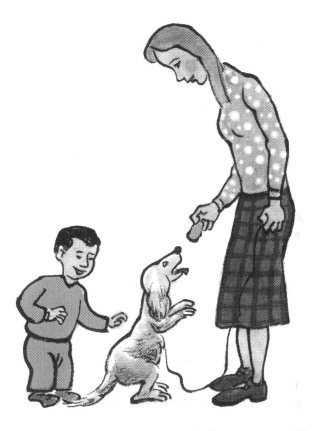

not the case. People with pets were physically not very different from people without pets, at least not in the general physical examination. Professor Friedman thus concluded that living with a pet they like is indeed helpful to the recovery of patients with heart disease, which can reduce the mortality rate of heart disease by about 3%. This figure means that out of nearly one million people in the United States who die of heart disease every year, 30,000 may well be able to recover if they keep a pet! The latest research by Professor Adelson of Australia's Baker Medical Research Institute also proves that raising small animals is beneficial to health. Researchers have interviewed 5,741 patients with heart disease and asked them about their lifestyles and whether they had pets. They found that the blood cholesterol level of 784 patients who had pets was 20% lower than that of patients without pets, and calculated that this would reduce the mortality rate of heart disease by 4%. They also discovered that people accompanied by small animals had not only lower cholesterol levels but also lower blood lipid (triglyceride) levels and relatively normal blood pressure. Living a life with pets is equivalent to eating a low-salt diet or not drinking alcohol.

Why keeping pets is beneficial to health

Professor Sepal of the University of Pennsylvania and his team studied three groups of research participants with basically the same levels of health. One group was asked to keep dogs, the second was asked to keep cats, and the last group had no pets. One month later, the participants were examined and it was found that the level of health for participants with pets was significantly improved. Professor Sepal believes that there is special emotional support between people and pets, which is difficult to find between people. Although people use language to express their thoughts and feelings, sometimes they also use words to cheat and spread rumors, or criticize and verbally abuse. Pets, on the other hand, always listen silently and seem to understand, but never ask questions or make comments. They are loyal listeners and their silence is friendly rather than stressful, which produces some psychotherapeutic effect. Dogs and cats, in particular, are the most emotional and good at expressing unspoken feelings to people, making people feel appreciated, needed, admired and loved. Professor Sepal has pointed out, "People's self-confidence, self-esteem, ability to deal with life stress, and health level all depend on feelings, some of which can deeply support people to set up personal goals." People need a strong sense of responsibility while caring for small animals, which helps give profound meaning to life.

Naturally, there are also hidden dangers and problems when raising small animals. For example, dogs can bite people and spread parasitic diseases and rabies. Pigeons and parrots can cause lung infection. Cats can induce asthma. Turtles can spread salmonella. Pet feces can cause environmental pollution, etc. Therefore, for everyone who is reading and is considering keeping a pet, please don't forget that pets can also bring diseases. Please consider the pros and cons carefully before you decide to take on the responsibility of keeping a pet.

In this section, I have roughly talked about the significance of psychological balance to health, and how to achieve psychological balance. There are also many other ways to promote mental health in real life. Different people will encounter different situations at various stages. I hope everyone can adjust their mindsets in a timely and appropriate way based on their situation, so as to promote health.

"Work, love and leisure are three important aspects of life. If you neglect any of them, you cannot be counted as a mentally healthy person."

"When you are climbing a mountain, don't forget to enjoy the scenery around you."

Recently, I saw a post on the Internet and thought it was well written. We might as well give it a try:

Don't be angry. Anger can cause tumors, and you shouldn't torture yourself with other people's mistakes.

Don't worry about your children. Worry makes people age, let the children handle their own affairs.

Don't quarrel. If you are patient in one moment of anger, you will escape a hundred days of sorrow.

Be insensitive. Where ignorance is bliss, it's folly to be wise. A man of great wisdom often appears slow-witted.

Be optimistic. Think about good things and have fun.

Laugh more often. Laugh three times everyday and three minutes every time.

Balanced diet

Have a full breakfast (30%), a reasonable lunch (40%) and a rationed dinner (30%). The body needs to endure a bit of hunger and coldness to stay healthy. Diet should be "diversified." People should eat more vegetables and fruits of various colors, eat more white meat, limit the consumption of foods with high fat, especially animal fat, and limit their alcohol intake.

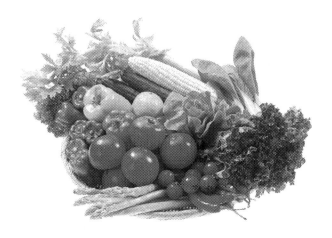

Bad eating habits are second only to smoking as a cause of cancer

Research by the American Cancer Society has pointed out that bad eating habits are second only to smoking as a carcinogenic factor. A series of epidemiology studies completed by Shanghai Cancer Institute show that eating too much pork, beef and mutton can increase the risk of colon cancer and kidney cancer. Excessive consumption of animal fat and protein can cause endometrial cancer and ovarian cancer. Eating too much food processed by pickling, smoking, sun drying, frying and other cooking methods is closely related to the occurrence of digestive tract cancers such as oropharynx, esophagus, stomach and pancreas cancer, as well as nasal cavity cancer and laryngeal cancer.

In fact, the number of calories people need on a daily basis is not a lot, and ordinary diets are enough. What I want to say is that there should not be too much fat in our diet, especially animal fat. There are more and more saturated fatty acids, that is, animal fat, in the diets of Chinese people, including children. It is extremely important to take in enough cellulose. The proportion of cellulose in whole grains, vegetables, fruits and other foods is relatively high. In recent years, colorectal cancer morbidity has been increasing in China and almost climbed to second place. The main reason for this is that the Chinese people's eating habits have changed greatly. Nowadays, Chinese people mainly eat refined grains that lack cellulose and cannot help intestinal peristalsis and digestion. Food that has stayed in the intestinal tract for too long will lead to constipation and produce harmful substances, leading to a sharp rise in the morbidity of colorectal cancer. Many cancers, including rectal cancer and colon cancer, are all related to alcohol consumption and the consumption of too much greasy food. Cellulose, which is needed everyday, is necessary for keeping the intestinal tract unobstructed.

We should also try to eat less junk food in daily life. Usually, food that only provides some energy and has no other nutrients, or that provides an excessive amount of nutrients that exceed the human body's demand and eventually become surplus substances in the human body, are called junk food. Fast food like McDonald's and KFC are the obvious examples. This kind of food contains more saturated fatty acids and it is better to eat as little of them as possible. In the United States, the increase of coronary disease morbidity in the blue-collar class is closely linked to bad eating habits. People eat fast food for various reasons, including time, convenience and of course, taste. The famous "fast-food mogul" Charlie Bell in the United States worked in McDonald's from an early age and was very hard-working. He became the chief executive officer of the company but died of colon cancer at the age of 44 because fast food was a big part of his diet.

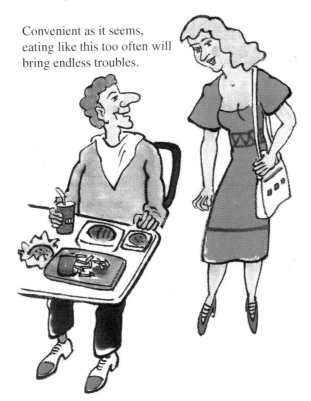

Convenient as it seems, eating like this too often will bring endless troubles.

Healthy eating habits are one of the most effective measures to prevent cancer

Recently, the World Cancer Research Fund invited 16 famous experts of oncology, nutriology, and epidemiology from 8 countries and comprehensively studied 45,000 pieces of the latest leading scientific research on diet and prevention of cancer in the world. Nearly 100 experts participated in writing and reviewing the research articles. After comprehensive analysis and argumentation, the summary report "Food, Nutrition, and the Prevention of Cancer" was published. The conclusion: preventing cancer through reasonable diet and physical activities is the most effective measure. Based on the cancer morbidity in 1996, the WHO estimated that the total number of cancer cases that could be prevented through dietary measures could reach 3–4 million per year. Due to the trend of dietary changes, population growth and aging, this number may reach 4.5 million to 6 million by 2025, which is 2–7 times that of cancer prevention through tobacco control. We can see from here how important healthy eating habits are.

Thus, the WHO proposed to prevent cancer by changing eating habits and introduced a dietary guide in 1996, which has been in use ever since. Years of efforts of adjusting eating habits have made more and more Americans realize that healthy eating habits are conducive to their health. It has also enabled more and more Americans to have the physical conditions to resist cancer. Research has discovered that many dietary components can induce apoptosis (programmed cell death), antioxidants in some foods can inhibit spontaneous mutation of cells, and about 1/3 of deaths of cancer patients can be avoided with feasible dietary methods.

Scientific eating habits are:

1. Have a full breakfast (30%).
2. Have a reasonable lunch (40%).
3. Have a rationed dinner (30%).

In terms of diet, I personally do not place too much emphasis on which kinds of food to eat. The statement that "any food sources that have four legs are not as good as those that have two legs" is not very scientific. What I strongly recommend is that the three meals in the morning, noon and evening should be distributed according to the ratio of 3:4:3. Besides, it should be emphasized that the dietary components should include protective nutrition, such as vitamins, plant pigments and dietary fiber. I myself have such a diet. When I say one should have a full breakfast, I do not mean that one should feel very full after breakfast. However, people must not miss breakfast and should also have a reasonably filling lunch. Then, for dinner, people should generally eat less.

But what is our diet like in reality? "I will skip breakfast, make do for lunch, and eat as much as I can for dinner." In particular, our friends from the business world treat guests, drink alcohol, and eat their fill at night. Then they skip breakfast and lunch the next day, which greatly affects their health. Socializing in the evenings may be necessary for their jobs, but people should properly control themselves. They should control their appetite, and never feel free to drink and eat whatever they want at night. Why? Because the stomach and intestines need to rest after a long day, if they have to work overtime instead, it is not good for health.

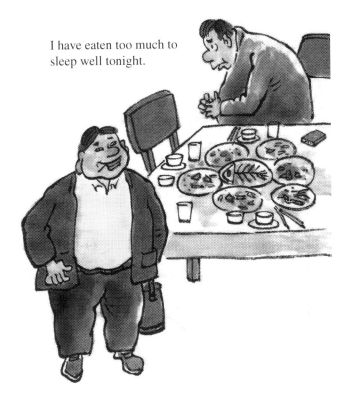

I have eaten too much to sleep well tonight.

There is another eating habit that I insist on very much: "The body needs to endure a bit of hunger and coldness to stay healthy." People should not eat too much, and 70%–80% full is the healthiest way. This is very important. If a person feels hungry and has a good appetite at every meal, then his/her digestive system is healthy and it is a good thing. However, the most harmful thing to the digestive system is when one eat too much for one meal and then loses appetite for several meals after that. Many people with long life spans have their own eating habits, and some of them are not conducive to health from a scientific point of view, such as eating fatty meat, smoking, drinking, etc. However, these long-lived people insist on one same thing, that is, don't overeat, and only eat until you feel 70%–80% full. This is very important if you want to stay healthy. Pay attention to the foods that you really enjoy. For example, when Chinese people from the north return to their hometowns and meet with family and friends, in addition to drinking, they have a competition of who can eat more dumplings. If one eats 50 dumplings, the other will eat 100 dumplings. This is too much for the stomach and intestine to recover even over a few days.

There was once a famous clinical mouse experiment. The mice were divided into two groups. One group was classifed as low energy and the other group high energy. The so-called high energy means that the mice were fed till they were very full and low energy means the mice were not fully fed and were often semi-hungry. The results showed that the lifespan of the high-energy group was 30% shorter than that of the low-energy group. In other words, the mice who ate their fill at each meal lived 30% shorter lives than mice that were not fully fed. Moreover, the prevalence rate of tumors was also lower in the low-energy group. It was because the excessive amounts of food had provided lots of oxides, saturated fatty acids, and other substances that largely exceeded the needs of the body and did great harm. Clinical medical research shows that the situation for humans is very similar.

My diet method

The general principle of a reasonable diet is: diet should be "diversified." People should eat more vegetables and fruits of various colors, eat more white meat, limit the consumption of high-fat food, especially animal fat, and limit alcohol intake.

As mentioned, the three meals of a day are distributed according to the ratio of 3:4:3.

Well, I eat four meals a day instead of three. The extra meal is a small snack at night. I have some basic principles for my four meals each day: First, don't eat too much. I only eat until I feel 70%–80% full at every meal. Second, eat more vegetables and fish. I always like fish. Third, do not choose or avoid any food deliberately, and eat a variety of food. I also eat fast food and McDonald's. But I only eat them occasionally, hence I think I can guarantee enough nutrition in general. Apart from eating fish and vegetables, I seldom eat animal fat, except for lean meat.

I take breakfast very seriously and never skip it. Many people are used to not having breakfast or casually eating a little, which does not meet their physiological needs. They must cultivate a habit of eating breakfast. This is really not easy for working people, because there is not much time in the morning. I only became accustomed to it after several years of training. My breakfast recipe often changes, including many different kinds of food, such as milk, porridge, toast, eggs, etc. My breakfast comprises at least 30% of the recommended daily calorie intake.

I usually have a small snack before bed, after a light dinner. I don't eat a lot. I just have a glass of milk and a few biscuits. Some women worry that they will get fat after eating food late at night. The key is to do so in moderation. It is best to eat two hours before going to bed and avoid inappropriate food with high fat, such as instant noodles, fried dough sticks and cakes. Greasy food will slow down digestion and delay gastric emptying, resulting in poor sleep at night and obesity. The better choices for late-night snacks are a cup of low-fat milk with two or three slices of lightly salted crackers, light noodles in soup or savory porridge, oatmeal, etc.

I don't like to stop to eat when I am busy at work. I prefer to delay the mealtime. I arrange four meals a day as follows: breakfast at 7:30 in the morning, lunch at 1:00 in the afternoon, dinner after 7:30, and something to eat before going to bed at 11:00. The time interval between two meals during the day is long, which aims to ensure that the stomach is emptied before the next meal. Although a person can feel satisfied if he/she eats a lot when hungry, it is not ideal for the stomach and the body. I have learnt about this fact from personal experience. In the past, I ate as much as I could when I liked the food, and eating too much led to gastric ulcer. Now I have changed my eating habits, and my gastric ulcer has healed. I have concluded that if I do not feel like eating a meal, then I must have been too full at the previous meal. If I feel hungry and want to eat, then I have eaten the right amount at the meal before.

A diversified diet is good for health

A diversified diet is good for health. It includes a mixture of all or most of the traditional food groups, such as vegetables, fruit, grains, meat, fish and dairy products. Nutrition experts suggest that eating 30 or more different kinds of food in a week or more than 12 types of food in a day is the ideal diet for the intake of basic nutrients. In this way, the potential positive and negative interactions between ingredients in food can be balanced, which enables nutrients of different forms in different food to balance the nutrients in human body in general. At the same time, a variety of food can increase people's interest in the diet.

However, I think this is somewhat dogmatic. It is difficult for ordinary people to comply, or they do not know how to do it and feel lost. My suggestion is that we eat from a variety of food groups.

Vegetables: onions, spinach, carrots, pumpkins, tomatoes, cruciferous vegetables, etc.
Fruit: apples, oranges, mangoes, etc.
Grains: corn, buckwheat, millet, rice and oats, etc.
Beans: soybeans, mung beans, etc.
Fungi: Jew's ear, mushrooms e.g. shitake.
Meat: fish, chicken, duck, pork, beef, etc.
Beverages: soy milk, yogurt, milk, green tea, etc.

The health benefits of these foods are common knowledge and easily obtainable from mass media coverage, so I will not talk much about them. I will mainly talk about a matter of principle in diet, that is, the diet should be diversified, balanced, and with proper combinations.

Most people want to implement a healthy diet, but the identification of the best diet is a big challenge. A lot of the information they have obtained through family, friends and mass media is contradictory, which makes people confused. I want to point out a simple way, which is to know which foods belong in each group and eat more high-quality and healthy food from each group. Nevertheless, you should not deliberately avoid certain foods or be too picky about food. As the saying goes, "Everything has its pros and cons." The same is true for food. There is no perfect food or worthless food. For example, fried food is commonly recognized as unhealthy, but it also has its own advantages. It is crispy and delicious, has a fragrant aroma, can stimulate appetite, partially supply human body with oil and fat-soluble vitamins, so it is okay in moderation. The intake of any food can have a certain degree of benefits, and no matter how much nutrition a kind of food has or how perfect it is, excessive intake will also bring harm. Therefore, it is not that we must not eat junk food at all. The key is to know how to balance one's nutrition, calories and diet, and how to reduce or avoid the harm of junk food to the body.

For example, if pregnant women only eat food that contains calcium to supplement calcium, they may end up with too much calcium and too little of some other nutrients, which is not ideal. If they eat food rich in vitamin D at the same time, it will be beneficial and can multiply the result of calcium absorption. Stewed beef with potatoes can not only reduce the greasiness of beef but also provide nutrition from both potatoes and beef. So, people can obtain various nutritional ingredients at the same time.

Choosing a variety of food everyday should also conform to another important piece of nutritional advice: "Aim at balance and moderation." A balanced diet includes adequate but not excessive intake of various nutrients and food types. For example, protein-rich foods, such as red meat, fish, poultry and livestock, are good sources of iron, but are not ideal sources of calcium. Milk and dairy products are high-quality protein-rich foods, rich in calcium but lacking iron. Therefore, in the daily diet, the regular intake of these two food groups is a good way to achieve a balanced calcium and iron supplement.

The concept of moderation and balance, and diversified diets complement each other. For example, the moderate intake of fat is the most fundamental requirement for a healthy diet, because sufficient fat (about 15% of the total energy contained in the diet) is very important to health. However, excessive intake may lead to obesity and heart disease. Based on this idea, the occasional consumption of high-fat foods can diversify the diet without sacrificing the quality of a healthy eating, especially when there are various kinds of fats and oils. Therefore, I eat almost everything. Apart from vegetables, fruit, fish, milk, and beans, I also eat a small amount of animal meat, including some animal fat.

Things to notice when eating meat

Nutrition science usually divides meat into red meat and white meat. Red meat refers to beef, pork, mutton, etc., as well as sausages, hamburger beef patties and smoked, vulcanized and salted meat (like ham and bacon) that are all processed with red meat. White meat mainly refers to fish, chicken and duck. As advised by many nutrition and health experts, more and more people nowadays know that there are things to notice when eating meat. They should eat less red meat and more white meat, and it is better not to eat salted, smoked, or barbecued meat. The reason is that white meat such as chicken, duck and fish contain less saturated fatty acids than red meat such as beef, pork, and mutton.

A six-year study led by Professor Walter at Harvard University revealed that women who eat about 150 grams of red meat a day have a 150% higher risk of colon cancer than women who eat less than 25 grams of red meat a day, and the risk of cancer increases with the growing consumption of red meat! Laboratory studies have proven that the chemicals formed in cooked meat have carcinogenic effects on the breasts and colon of rodents. In the process of roasting, baking and frying, the meat will produce a variety of chemicals on its surface, which are known carcinogens. A British epidemiological investigation believes that meat intake is indeed related to an increased risk of breast cancer. Many research data have proven that the large consumption of meat (especially red meat) and processed meat is a positive risk factor for colorectal cancer, prostate cancer and pancreatic cancer. Researchers at the University of Northern California have found that young people who eat hot dogs at least once a week are twice as likely to develop brain tumors as those who do not eat hot dogs. Additionally, young people who like to eat other smoked and salted red meat (such as ham, bacon and sausags) are 80% more likely to suffer from brain tumors.

Buy some white meat and try to eat
less cured meat.

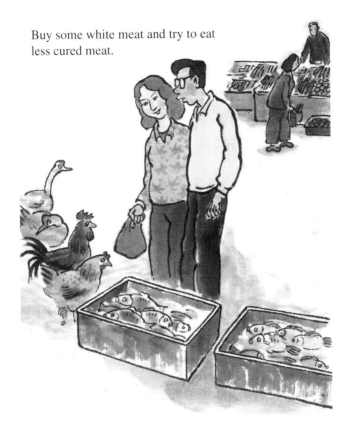

Recently, two major nutrition reports in Britain suggest that people's intake of red meat or processed meat should be reduced, or at least not increased. The report of the World Cancer Research Fund recommends that if red meat is inevitable in the diet, it should provide less than 1/10 of the total daily intake of calories (i.e., the daily intake of red meat should be limited to less than 100 grams). The most effective way is to replace red meat with white meat. I suggest that people eat more fish. The meat of fish is tender and easier to digest and absorb than livestock meat and poultry. It is especially suitable for children and the elderly. Meanwhile, fish has less fat and its unsaturated fatty acids account for 80% of the total fat, which is of great benefit to the prevention and treatment of cardiovascular diseases. The Omega-3 polyunsaturated fatty acids in fish meat can inhibit the growth of malignant tumors. Animal experiments conducted by Dr. Roebuck at Geisel School of Medicine at Dartmouth show that feeding animals with Omega-3 will reduce the risk of pancreatic cancer. Dr. Danenberg, director of the Strang Cancer Prevention Institute in New York, has pointed out that the Omega-3 fatty acid in fish can stimulate the action of enzymes in the detoxification mechanism of the body. American Professor Walter's research has indicated that eating fish 2–4 times a day can reduce the risk of intestinal cancer by 25%.

Cook properly and have a balanced diet

I have mentioned above about eating more white meat and less red meat, but it does not mean going to the other extreme — completely refusing red meat. The key is to eat in a healthy way. Red meat does contain more saturated fat than white meat, but it is not necessarily harmful. It can provide abundant nutrients. Red meat is rich in minerals, particularly iron. Chinese people, especially women, generally suffer from severe iron deficiency. Thus, eating red meat can help achieve the purpose of supplementing iron.

It is all about balance.

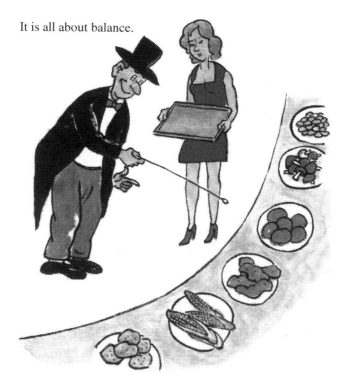

People must have saturated and unsaturated fatty acids to survive. Unsaturated fatty acids can be used to adjust various functions of the human body. It can help dispose of redundant "garbage" in the human body, which is the extra fat formed after the intake of too much saturated fatty acids. If the human body lacks unsaturated fatty acids, a series of changes will occur in all aspects of its functions. First, prostaglandins PGE1-PGE3 cannot be synthesized, which will cause prostate inflammation. Second, the immune, cardiovascular and cerebrovascular, reproductive, endocrine and other systems will become abnormal and out of balance, thus leading to a series of diseases such as hyperlipidemia, high blood pressure, thrombosis, atherosclerosis, rheumatism, diabetes, rough skin, accelerated aging, etc. Many people suffer from these diseases without any reason in their life, and do not know the cause. The fundamental cause is the lack of unsaturated fatty acids in their body.

A research by Harvard University has proven that the "culprit" resulting in the increase of blood lipids and harmful cholesterol is not natural fat found in food, but unhealthy processing methods, such as frying and over-refining of flour and sugar. Unsaturated fat has an unstable character and is easy to oxidize, especially when treated at high temperature. The lipids and bad cholesterol in the blood are caused by the accumulation of solidified substances formed after fat is oxidized. Although white meat contains more unsaturated fat than red meat, in high-temperature cooking such as frying and microwaving, the free radicals generated after the unsaturated fat is oxidized are toxins that are able to turn its positive nutritional value into negative value.

Therefore, meat and other food should be cooked processed as little as possible by salting, smoking, roasting, and frying. Methods like steaming and stewing can be adopted. Meat cooked using these methods produces fewer carcinogens. Meanwhile, we should also pay attention to the balance of meat and vegetables, and not overeat.

When boiling and stewing, we should eat the meat as well as drink the soup. Some people mistakenly believe that drinking soup is the best way to fully absorb the nutrients in the meat. However, most of the nutrients in the meat do not come out of the tissue cells into the soup in stewing. If we only drink soup but not eat the meat, it will be like putting the cart before the horse.

Have a proper supplement of vitamins and micronutrients

In recent years, vitamins have become a hot topic again. In February 2007, the American Medical Association, published a research jointly completed by researchers from many countries. The study showed that the mortality rate of those taking vitamin E had increased by 4%, mortality rate of those taking carotene had increased by 7%, and mortality rate of those taking vitamin A had increased by 16%. However, there was no evidence that vitamin C can prolong life expectancy. Domestic media in China reported the research, causing quite a stir. At that time, various points of views were advanced and the ordinary people became confused. Personally, I think that the American research has shown that too many vitamins can cause side effects, but Chinese people should take vitamins according to our current dietary habits and the differences between regions and urban and rural areas. I have been taking multivitamins for 35 years. I believe this is the only way to ensure adequate vitamin intake.

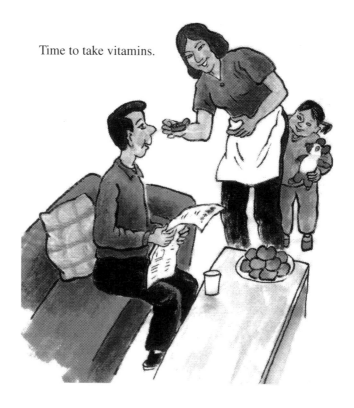

Time to take vitamins.

Quit smoking and limit alcohol consumption

Smoking can cause more than 40 fatal diseases, including oral cancer, esophageal cancer, laryngeal cancer, lung cancer and gastric cancer. Most human tissues, organs and systems can be affected by smoking. Indeed, up to 3 million deaths are caused by smoking-related diseases globally each year (one death in every ten seconds). To make it worse, this figure is expected to reach 10 million in 2020.

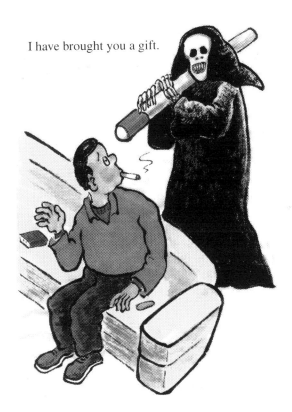

I have brought you a gift.

Smoking is a health hazard

The dangers of tobacco have become one of the most serious public issues in the world today, and it is also the biggest problem facing human health. Smoking is also a very significant problem in China. At present, China has the dubious honor of ranking first in the world with regard to the production of tobacco and cigarettes, and the number of smokers. According to statistics, the rate of men over 15 years old in China who smoke is 53%, and that of women is close to 5%. There are as many as 300 million smokers, accounting for a quarter of the 1.1 billion smokers in the world. A large number of studies have proven that the smoke generated by cigarettes contains more than 4,000 chemicals, and 69 of them are carcinogens. Some of them are also the components of varnish, the pesticide DDT, poisons, nail polish remover and rat poison. Almost all human tissues, organs or systems can be negatively influenced by smoking. Among them, the most sensitive parts are the respiratory system, circulatory system, nervous system and digestive system. Certainly, the immune system is also very likely to be damaged by smoking. If people smoke for a long period of time, the ash, tar, harmful gases and other toxins contained in cigarettes will damage their bodies, hearts and lungs, cause their senses of taste and smell to degenerate, and weaken their ability to resist infection.

Smoking is harmful to health, and everyone knows it. But why has it not been completely banned? Many people who have failed to quit smoking or do not want to quit delude themselves by saying that "a cigarette after a meal is better than the life of a god." They also claim that smoking can enhance memory, sharpen thinking, adjust emotions and even improve work efficiency. At the time of SARS, many people even believed that "smoking can prevent SARS infection." Admittedly, some substances contained in tobacco, such as nicotine, may generate some "feel good" effects after inhalation, but the disadvantages of smoking far outweigh any "benefits."

More than 20 years ago, people used to see giant billboards like the one below on TV or in public places such as railway stations.

They featured a cool young man with deep eyes and brown skin, dressed in jeans, and smoking a cigarette on a red steed. He was the spokesperson of Marlboro who converted a large number of boys and girls to smoking. But unfortunately, he died of lung cancer before he was 60 years old. Before his death, he spoke from his heart: "I am killed by cigarettes. It is not worthy to die for cigarettes. Tell the children that they should never smoke cigarettes!"

Some people say that Deng Xiaoping smoked until he was 92 years old. In fact, he was already coughing badly in his 80s. More than a dozen of doctors advised him not to smoke anymore. He asked, "Is smoking really that harmful?" The doctors answered with one voice: "Yes!" He said, "Well, then I will stop smoking." Then he put out his cigarette and the next day he really stopped smoking. After smoking for decades, it was surprising that he had the ability to quit as soon as he wanted to.

Smoking and lung cancer

Since it is my area of expertise, I will put focus more on smoking and lung cancer in this section. In the early 1980s, the lung cancer morbidity among men in Britain, Germany and the United States began to rise. At that time, medical professionals had put forward various reasons, but they did not think that smoking was a critical reason. They only focused on the dust on asphalt roads, gas pollution from factories and smoke from coal burning. In the 1990s, the international medical community successively published the results of five extensive case-control studies, all of which showed that smoking was closely connected to lung cancer. At the same time, the *British Journal of Oncology* published a famous research article. The study involved 50 years of observation and comparison of the tumor morbidity of three groups of people, including those who did not smoke, those who had quit smoking and those who were still smoking. It was found that the number of cigarettes smoked per day is entirely proportional to multiple tumors. The more one smokes, the higher the morbidity of tumors. In particular, the prevalence rate of lung cancer has increased by 10–20 times, laryngeal cancer by 6–10 times, and coronary disease by 2–3 times, all of which are very significant (see the table on the next page). Based on the analysis of these facts, the study concluded that the increase in tobacco consumption in the past half century likely accounts for and explains the sharp increase in the number of lung cancer patients in many countries. Currently, the number of people who die of smoking-related diseases worldwide is as high as 3 million each year, which is equivalent to one death every 10 seconds. Experts have estimated that this number could rise to 10 million by 2020.

A survey was conducted in Shanghai about the correlation between male smokers and deaths by malignant tumors in urban areas. The study followed more than 18,000 male residents (aged 45–64), the researchers conducted follow-up visits once a year, and found that 419 people died of lung cancer. Furthermore, with the increasing number of cigarettes smoked, the morbidity of lung cancer also gradually increased. The conclusion was that the morbidity of lung cancer is closely related to smoking. If one does not smoke, the fatality rate of lung cancer will be 43.5%/100,000. But, the percentage of smokers (more than one pack per day) is 411.7%/100,000, a difference of nearly ten times. This survey was conducted over a span of 13 years. It has a large sample size and shows clearly that smoking is an important cause of deaths of lung cancer among middle-aged and elderly men in Shanghai urban areas.

In 1990, a prospective scientific study was conducted in Britain to investigate the rate of cumulative death risk by lung cancer among men at different ages (until 75 years old) after quitting smoking. Research results

Table 5: Correlation between smoking and tumor mortality rate [Person/(Year · 100,000)].

(British doctors' observation of deaths by tumor in the past 50 years)

Tumor types	Number of deaths	Non-smokers	Cigarette smokers					Other smokers	
			Ex-smokers	Current smokers	Number of cigarettes smoked per day			Ex-smokers	Current smokers
					1–14	15–24	≥25		
Oral cancer	13	19	13	7.1	4	3.7	15.9	4.4	6.8
Larynx cancer	40	0	2.6	10.3	6	8.5	17.3	2.9	4.7
Lung cancer	1052	16.9	68.8	249	130.6	233.8	415.2	69.8	129.8
Esophagus cancer	207	5.7	20.1	34.4	21.2	34.4	50	18.9	25.1
Stomach cancer	324	28.1	25.4	41.9	38.5	47.6	38.8	28.1	37.5
Pancreatic cancer	272	20.6	30.5	39.4	37.9	31.3	52.9	15.9	32.1
Kidney cancer	140	9.3	13.2	16.2	16.4	16.6	15.5	12.1	18.2
Bladder cancer	220	13.7	22.6	38.8	37.7	31.8	51.4	14.5	24.5
Liver cancer	74	4.4	5.7	13.6	10.7	2.6	31.3	8.1	8.3

showed that with the increase of the age of smoking cessation, the fatality rate of lung cancer also increased. In other words, the later you quit smoking, the higher the risk of onset of lung cancer (see figure below).

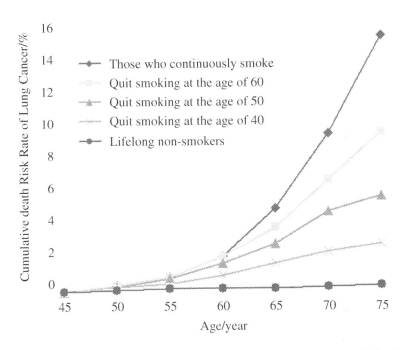

Correlation between smoking cessation age and rate of cumulative death risk by lung cancer.

Studies in China have also shown that the total prevalence rate of chronic obstructive pulmonary disease (COPD) among male smokers is one time higher than that among non-smokers and two times higher than that among women. If people who have COPD still smoke, their lung function will degenerate sharply. Within five to ten years, they will have symptoms such as shortness of breath after activities.

Even a little second-hand smoke is dangerous

Non-smokers are passively smoking when exposed to cigarette smoke for more than 15 minutes a day. The dangers of active smoking are well known to all, but the harmfulness of passive smoking is often ignored.

People always think that if they don't smoke, smoking won't hurt them, but it is not true. According to a recent report published by authoritative researchers in the United States, passive smoking (commonly known as "second-hand smoking") is more harmful than what people believe. Second-hand smoke can cause non-smokers to have cancer, respiratory problems and heart diseases. People affected by second-hand smoke are more likely to suffer from the common cold and flu. They have a shorter life expectancy than people not affected by second-hand smoke.

Close contacts, i.e., the relatives and friends of smokers, are the ones most affected by second-hand smoke. Statistics from Britain show that the number of cigarettes smoked by a person was proportional to the number of tumors their spouse had. In particular, the morbidity of lung cancer and adenocarcinoma (cancer beginning in glandular cells) increased evidently. Women living with their husbands or boyfriends who were smokers were 40% more likely to suffer from cervical cancer than women whose spouses did not smoke. Experts found in experiments that for both smoking and non-smoking women, they had a large amount of cotinine, the metabolite of nicotine, agglutinated on their uterine mucosa. It indicates clearly that non-smoking women are also negatively affected when living in a smoky environment.

Second-hand smoke can also endanger the health of newborn babies. Research by British experts show that if one of the parents is a "smoker", it is as if their children are "smoking." Futhermore, even the parents' clothes are the source of second-hand smoke for their babies. Research results show that if parents smoke at home, the content of the metabolite of nicotine, cotinine, in their children's urine is 5.58 times that of newborns from "smoke-free" families on average. If these babies usually sleep with their parents, then the content of cotinine in their bodies is even higher. It may be well because they have more contact with their parents' clothes that have the smell of smoke.

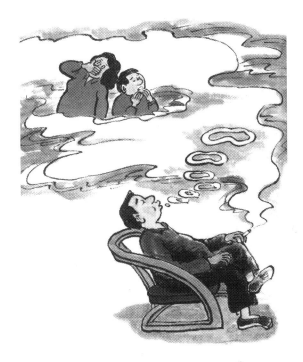

I strongly disapprove of smoking. In the United States, smoking has been banned in most public places, which has led to a continuous decline in the number of smokers. Correspondingly, the morbidity of lung cancer in the United States began to show a downward trend since the 1990s. Nevertheless, the numbers for the onset of lung cancer in females began to rise, which was consistent with the pattern that the number of male smokers decreased while the number of female smokers increased. Regardless, 1/4 of the 300 million people in the United States still smoke, although they know that smoking may lead to diseases such as lung cancer, heart disease and stroke. In response, Severin, the director-general of a Cancer Prevention Society in the United States, said, "We have reached the time when we must strengthen anti-smoking education." Many experts agree with this view: quitting smoking is not only beneficial to oneself but also beneficial for the health of family members. After quitting smoking for 1–2 years, the atypical changes of epithelial cells in the respiratory tract are inclined to reverse to healthy cells. After five years, the morbidity of lung cancer will decrease significantly, and it will be similar to that of non-smokers after 15 years.

Quit smoking today

I have met some patients with lung cancer clinically. The onset of their lung cancer happened after they had quit smoking for a year or two. They thought quitting smoking was the cause of lung cancer because they often felt uncomfortable after they stopped smoking. Their appetite and sleep were also affected. They felt that it was better when they still smoked, as they were able to eat and sleep normally and not get sick. This idea is completely wrong. An American report has shown that the average mortality rate of smokers is 10.8 times that of ex-smokers and that the lung cancer morbidity of those start smoking in their teenage years is about twice that of smokers who start after the age of 25. According to the investigation and statistical analysis of ex-smokers, after stopping smoking for 2–10 years, the risk of lung cancer is still about 8 times higher than that of non-smokers and 2.2 times higher than that of those who have quit smoking for more than 10 years. Other investigations and studies have pointed out that after smoking cessation, the morbidity of lung cancer can be significantly reduced and can reach the level of non-smokers after 15 years of quitting smoking.

There are many benefits of smoking cessation. Consider this: I will immediately feel healthier. My teeth will be whiter. My breath will be fresher and I will cough less. I will have more money to use. In my lifetime, I will have a lower risk of cancer, stroke, premature death and skin wrinkling. I will set a correct example for my children. No more people will be exposed to second-hand smoke because of me …

For those who are interested in quitting smoking, I can introduce the following method, it will definitely bring good results.

First, remind your relatives and friends that you want to quit smoking immediately. Invite them to support you, encourage you and help you overcome the difficulties in the first few days and weeks.

Stay busy. (1) Keep your daily schedule full. You may watch movies, play ball games, walk long distances, ride a bicycle, etc. (2) Try to spend your spare time in places where smoking is forbidden, such as shopping malls, libraries, museums or theatres. (3) When you can't help but want to hold a cigarette in your hand, try to hold other things, such as a pen, a ball or a cup. (4) Drink more water and juice. Avoid drinking alcohol, which can easily encourage you to smoke.

Avoid triggers. Don't smoke after meals. Stand up, brush your teeth or go for a walk. Do things that make you unable to smoke. Go to places where smoking is forbidden, and if you have to go to places that make you want to smoke (parties or bars), please stay with non-smokers (remember that most people do not smoke).

Make plans to reward yourself. Quitting smoking saves money. You can make a list and then use the saved "cigarette money" to buy the things on the list. You can also buy something for yourself to celebrate. Of course, more importantly, within 20 minutes after smoking, toxic gases and nicotine begin to leave your body, and your pulse and the oxygen in your blood return to normal levels. Within a few days, you will find that your ability to taste and smell improves, you breathe better, and the "smoke cough" slowly disappears.

Find something new to do. Make some new habits from the first day of quitting smoking. You can try the following things:

Exercise. Take time out everyday to exercise or join fitness groups. Exercise can not only divert your attention but also consume calories, helping you control your weight. The exercise can be swimming, running, playing tennis, or cycling.

Don't leave your hands idle. You can do jigsaw puzzles or try sewing, make some small handicrafts, work in the garden or do housework.

Enjoy the clean feeling in your mouth. Brush your teeth regularly and use mouthwash.

When you want to take out a cigarette and smoke, stand up and move around instead.

Resist the temptation, and do not be afraid of setbacks. Quitting smoking is not easy. Many ex-smokers try many times before they succeed. If you were not able to resist the temptation at the beginning and smoked one or two cigarettes, don't lose heart or blame yourself too much. A few setbacks don't mean failure or inability to quit smoking forever. However, don't be too lenient on yourself. When encountering setbacks, don't say "I have smoked anyway. I will just finish this whole pack." Instead, you should immediately stop smoking.

Moderate drinking is not for everyone

The description of alcohol in traditional Chinese medicine is: "It promotes blood circulation. It can remove one's sorrow and make one happy. If one drinks a little alcohol, it will strengthen the spirit. Drinking too much will hurt one's health." Usually, after moderate drinking, one's heartbeat is accelerated and blood flow will speed up. So, when the weather is cold, alcohol can stabilize the intestines and stomach, prevent one from getting a cold, and promote blood circulation. For a long time, it has been believed that moderate drinking is good for health. Researchers from the Institute on Aging of the University of Florida in Gainesville also believe that the elderly who drink moderately have a lower probability of cardiovascular diseases. They collected information from 2,500 elderly people aged 70 to 79, of which none had suffered from any type of heart disease, half did not drink at all, and the rest were moderate drinkers. Researchers followed these people for five and a half years, during which 307 people died and 383 developed heart diseases. They found that those who drank seven times a week had a 27.4% lower death probability and a 29% lower risk of heart disease than the teetotalers.

However, this kind of universal affirmation of moderate drinking has recently been questioned. A new study released by scientists at the University of California shows that in some cases, drinking two cups of alcohol a week increases the risk of death for some elders. Elderly people who drink moderately or heavily, if suffering from some other diseases such as gout or ulcer, or taking some drugs that can have an adverse interaction with alcohol, face a 20% higher risk of death than those who drink little or no alcohol but do not have the above diseases.

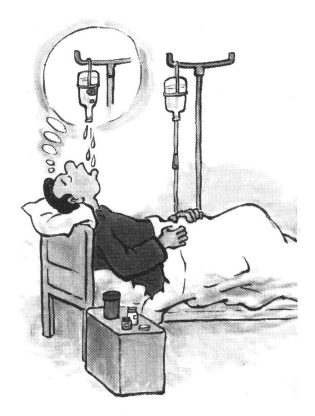

I believe that the research about moderate drinking reducing the occurrence of cardiovascular diseases and the mortality rate caused by cardiovascular diseases has not considered the possible adverse reactions that result from interaction between alcohol and other diseases or drugs. Moderate drinking may be a healthy choice for the elderly who have no other diseases. However, for those who need to take some commonly used drugs, such as sleeping pills and joint analgesics, or those suffering from depression and gastrointestinal diseases, drinking can have some unsafe consequences. Therefore, the benefits to health from moderate drinking vary from person to person and cannot be generalized.

However, what is certain is that excessive drinking or even binge drinking is harmful to the body.

Alcohol is a kind of pure energy food, and the energy it contains is relatively high. If one drinks too much, and takes in too much energy, other nutrients will not be absorbed by the body. Therefore, it is easy for drinkers to suffer from a lack of protein, minerals and vitamins. For example, the lack of electrolyte potassium and magnesium can affect the heart and nerves, and the neurological symptoms of alcoholism are more serious. As people take in a large amount of water while drinking alcohol, the excretion of the kidney will increase, and a large number of vitamins and minerals will be excreted from the kidney, thus making the above nutrients even more scarce. Alcohol affects appetite and irritates the digestive system. It can stimulate gastrointestinal mucosa, causing mucosal hyperemia, which leads to acute gastritis. Due to the long-term stimulation of alcohol, tongue vessels will become cancerous and chronic gastritis and enteritis will easily emerge. Drinking a large amount of strong liquor will lead to acute pancreatitis. Long-term drinking will lead to chronic pancreatitis, which will prevent the pancreas from secreting digestive enzymes and form chronic diarrhea, resulting in poor nutrient absorption. Alcohol can affect the central nervous system and the autonomic nervous system. Drinkers are very prone to neuroses, such as headache, sweating, amnesia, vertigo and even schizophrenia-like symptoms. After alcohol is absorbed into the liver, it can directly act on liver parenchymal cells, causing symptoms similar to fatty liver. If one drinks too much for a long time, it will evolve into fatty liver, and become liver cirrhosis if aggravated.

Proper exercise

When you regard physical exercise and functional exercise as indispensable and important components of life like eating, working and sleeping, your spiritual level will reach a new height.

In my dictionary of health, I have kept a word for decades, that is, exercise. When I was studying in Beijing Medical College, I trained in track and field. I believe my good physique is built on the foundation laid then. Although I have left the competition field now, I do all sorts of sports like basketball, running, swiming... I play basketball on Fridays and badminton on Sundays. Even if I am busy, as long as I have 10 minutes, I will take the time to exercise. For example, I run at home, and my treadmill is beside the bed in my bedroom.

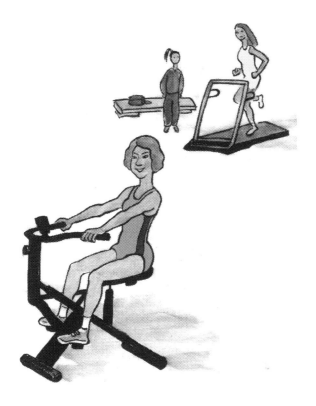

Swedish scientists conducted a 12-year follow-up survey of 3,206 people over 65 years old and found that regular exercise once or twice a week can prolong life expectancy, and the exercise included cycling and walking. If people exercise occasionally, they may reduce their risk of death by 28%. And exercising every week may reduce the risk of death by up to 40%. The study also found that exercising more than once or twice a week cannot increase the rate beyond 40%.

However, there is a misconception in many people's minds. They think that they can achieve the goal of exercise by playing ball games, taking a walk, swimming, hiking and sweating it all out. In fact, we also need to pay attention to both physical fitness exercise and functional exercise. They are two different things.

Let's first look at a human being's physical condition from birth to 70 years old. From birth to the age of 30, the physical condition is on the rise and reaches a peak around age 30. At this time, people can take part in competitions and so on. After age 30, a person's physical condition begins to decline, and physical fitness exercise is needed. After the ages of 40 or 50, the physical condition begins to degenerate, and functional exercise is needed at this time.

These concepts are different from each other. So, what is physical fitness exercise? It is using some means of practice to enable the functional improvement of various systems of the human body. What functions? There are a few:

The first is strength, which includes muscle strength, function of bones and function of joints.

However, this has degenerated for many people of my age. They cannot stand straight, their arms become soft, and their muscles have shrunk.

The second is speed and agility, which represent a person's physiological reaction ability.

The third is endurance, which indicates a person's cardiopulmonary function, that is, function of a person's visceral organs, including mainly respiratory function and heart function.

The fourth is flexibility, which means a person's body coordination ability and is a type of advanced performance. Some people slip and break their bones. Some other people slip but their body positions when they fall allow them to get up and walk again. Why? Because they are flexible and have superior coordination function.

Let me give you an example of the principle of "use it or lose it." Shenzhou VI astronauts Fei Junlong and Nie Haisheng stayed in space for nearly 120 hours and were carried out when they left the cabin. Why? Because they were weightless in space. They had little leg movement, carried little weight, used little force, and they had "lost it" over time. Once they were on land, their muscle strength dropped by 2/3, bone weight decreased by 30%, and their legs lost function. If they had stood up, they would have broken their bones. The same is true for us. If we sit all day and do not move, when we try to conduct activities again, our limbs will not work properly.

The quality of a man's muscles is closely related to male hormones. For young adults, hormone secretion is abundant. Their bodies contain lots of muscle and little fat. After middle age, hormone secretion decreases. People have more fat and less muscle. In old age, there are fewer muscles, leaving only skin and bones. Such a process is the same for everyone. But how can one delay this process? It requires muscle exercise and physical fitness exercise. Both men and women are in need of it.

When a woman is born, she is cute. She will be graceful at eighteen or nineteen years old, full of charm in her twenties and thirties, and begin to fade in her forties or fifties. When menopause its, she will be fidgety and moody, and she will become old finally. This is the law of nature. But how can we slow down the process? It requires muscle movement.

We know that female hormone estrogen is essential, and the secretion of estrogen can make muscles, skin, and mammary glands, become plump and develop. Once estrogen secretion drops, all aspects of a person will begin to degenerate. Look at your loving mother or grandmother. She was quite tall when she was young, but when she is 70 or 80 years old, she would be ten centimeters shorter. Why? The answer is osteoporosis. According to statistics, 50% of the people over 50 years old in China suffer from osteoarthritis or osteoporosis. Cases of people over 65 years old are more serious, with 80% suffering from osteoarthritis. Women over 40 years old are in the worst situation because women's estrogen secretion begin to decrease after 40, leading to osteoporosis and fractures.

However, "degeneration" can be delayed through exercises of muscles and bones. Muscle movement can form benign vascular massage, maintaining elasticity and making it difficult for blood vessels to harden.

It's important to get all four types of exercise. Each one has different benefits. Doing one kind also can improve your ability to do the others. Strength is about the exercise of muscles and bones. Agility is about exercising the nervous system. Endurance is about aerobic metabolism, which works on lung and heart functions. Flexibility is about stretching your muscles and helping your body stay limber

Former California Governor Schwarzenegger was once a world champion in bodybuilding when he was young. But later he exercised less. By the age of 60, his muscles were loose, like walking with a bag.

When I was in Beijing Medical College, I was young and far from being able to compare with Schwarzenegger. At the age of 70, I was 10 years older than him, but I still had the physique of a young man and did not walk like him. Why? It is because I did muscle exercises. I still like swimming and playing basketball now.

In 1984, at the age of 48, I played basketball...

After SARS in 2003, I was 68 years old and played basketball...

After the 2006 Doha Asian Games, I was responsible for the last leg of the torch relay in Guangzhou.

Therefore, I strongly advise that everyone should have appropriate exercise. People should do a reasonable amount of exercise instead of exercising everyday until exhausted as if they were addicted.

There are many examples of deaths caused by extreme or excessive exercise:

As mentioned earlier, Jan Malm, former president of Beijing Ericsson (China) Communications Co., Ltd., went to the gym after returning to Beijing from a business trip to Shanghai and died on the treadmill. He died of sudden death at the age of 54.

Some newspaper once reported that a university teacher often slept at 1–2 a.m. and got up at 5 a.m. He was sleep-deprived for a long time. He also invigilate more than 30 exams in one semester. He did more than 100 push-ups in a row during exercise. As a result, he died of sudden cardiac death at the age of 46.

Walking is the best exercise in the world

If you are too tired, don't force yourself to exercise. You can take a walk and adjust the pace so it is comfortable for yourself. What's more important is it should be done in a scientific way. How? For working people and the elderly, aerobic exercise is indeed necessary. Aerobic exercise and anaerobic exercise are opposite. Aerobic exercise is not too strenuous exercise. Representative aerobic exercises include jogging, swimming, aerobics, mountaineering, cross-country walking, rope skipping, various ball games and brisk walking. These exercises can accelerate your heart rate, deepen your breathing, fully mobilize the body's movement and regulation potential. It can help discharge metabolic wastes from the body to the maximum extent with the acceleration of blood circulation and the deepening of breathing. Aerobic exercise is different from extreme exercise. Extreme exercise can be considered as a challenge to the physiological limits of the human body, such as the marathon, triathlon, cross-country race, etc. Normal people cannot complete it without professional training. Blind pursuit without preparation will do more harm than good and even damage the body. For example, the heart suddenly beats very fast during strenuous exercise, which is not suitable for people above middle age. People above middle age should do aerobic exercises

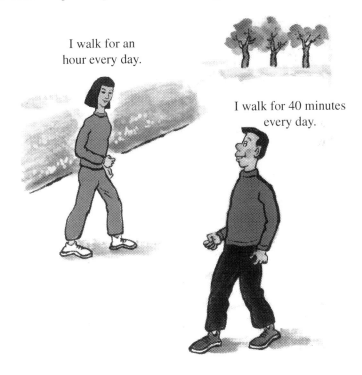

I walk for an hour every day.

I walk for 40 minutes every day.

that are gentle, comfortable and slow, allowing the heart rate to continuously increase over a period of time. This kind of exercise is suitable for them.

What exercise can people choose from this description? There are two kinds. One is the exercises that older men and women in their 70s and 80s usually do, such as Tai Chi. The other is what the WHO suggests, walking. For example, brisk walking. Brisk walking does not require special conditions and will not cause damage to bones and joints. When walking at a brisk pace, the distance between strides should be regular and people should touch the ground with their heels. In this way, it will produce some mechanical stimulation to bones. It has the characteristics of sports with impact, and can have positive effects on enhancing bone strength and preventing osteoporosis, and yet not make the heart beat irregularly. These effects are based on the prospective study that the WHO conducted of 1,645 people over 65 years old for more than four years. By comparing two groups of people who walked more than four hours and less than one hour per week, respectively, the results were surprising. The group walking more than 4 hours per week had 69% fewer cardiovascular morbidity and 73% fewer fatality than the group with less than 1 hour of walking per week. What an amazing difference!

I still keep running, but usually in the afternoon. Morning is not suitable for vast amounts of exercise, and one's biological clock is more accustomed to afternoon exercise. Do people have to exercise everyday? Not necessarily. It is enough to exercise about four times a week. My current exercise routine is usually like this: I run on the treadmill for about half an hour. I first walk fast, then run. The amount of exercise is based on heart rate. My basic heart rate is 60 beats/minute, and running to 120 beats/minute is enough for me. My age is suitable for doing aerobic exercise instead of anaerobic exercise. Thus, my heart rate cannot be too fast. I also do other sports with a relatively regular rhythm, such as swimming, gymnastics and pulling exercises.

The "good stature and poor physical fitness" of teenagers is worrying

The decline of teenagers' physical health has become an increasingly significant global problem, and similar situations have occurred successively in the United States, Japan, South Korea and other countries. According to the WHO's statistics, about 22 million children under the age of 5 are overweight worldwide. Type II diabetes among children and adolescents was unheard of in the past. However, such cases have begun to appear all over the world now. In Britain, the rate of overweight children aged 2–10 has increased from 23% in 1995 to 28% in 2003. In China, the numbers of overweight urban children are also on the rise, and foreign media have also started to focus on this problem. *USA Today* reported that the growth rate of obese children in China is as fast as that of China's economy, which has sparked concern that Chinese children are likely to encounter the problem of American-style obesity. The rapid development of China's economy has enriched the dining tables of Chinese families, and increasing wealth has also affected people's lifestyles. People do less manual labor, have fewer opportunities for walking or cycling, and frequently ride in a car and surf the Internet for long hours.

According to data from China's Ministry of Education, 8% of urban children aged 10 to 12 in China are considered obese, and 15% are overweight. These numbers are close to the relevant data of the United States. According to a 2006 report by the US Department of Health and Public Utilities, 18.8% of American children aged 6 to 11 are overweight. The *British Medical Journal* has stated that China is also catching up with the West in terms of the obesity issue. From 1985 to 2000, the number of obese children in China has increased 28 times.

Relevant departments report that the physical health of young people in our nation is on a continuous decline. Since 1985, China has conducted four national surveys on the physical health of young people. The results show that the physical health of Chinese teenagers has been declining in the past 20 years. Among the 300 million teenagers in the nation, more than 15% are obese or malnourished, which means that the number of them exceeds 45 million. The myopia rate of students exceeds 50% in the stage of junior high school, 76% in senior high school and 83% in university. The trend is absolutely shocking. The nutrition survey and analysis in 2002 showed that among the students aged 7–17, the morbidity risk, blood pressure, and risk factor of metabolic syndrome, high blood sugar, high blood pressure and coronary disease of obese and overweight children were higher than that of normal-weight children. Some experts have summed up the physical condition of teenagers as "stiff, soft and clumsy", which indicate that teenagers have stiff joints, soft muscles, and uncoordinated and clumsy movements caused by long-term inactivity. What worries people is that while the morphological development indexes such as height and weight of young people in the nation continue to increase, their physical qualities such as vital capacity, speed and strength continue to decline. According to a 2005 survey, the vital capacity of male and female young people aged 7–18 decreased by 300 mL (10%–15%) compared with the year of 2000, and the speed performance of standing long jump and 50 m running decreased significantly. It can be said that "good stature and poor physical fitness" have made Chinese teenagers "weaker than they look", and it is easy for the superficial phenomenon of being tall to cover up the reality of poor physique.

Adolescence is a sensitive period for the development and growth of adolescents. The physical fitness of this period determines the physical condition of one's life. If this period is compromised, one can never make up for it. Let's put it this way: when people are still students, their physical health is not able to have a significant impact on learning. Once they have started working, they have to face pressure from all aspects of life while also aging. The conditions of physical health play a vital role at that time. Teenagers should not just be satisfied with not being ill, because young people can live with some minor problems. But, not being ill does not mean being very healthy. Young people may not get sick even if they have poor physical conditions, but the harm will gradually appear in their middle age. Therefore, both parents and society should have a long-term vision.

Be as vigorous as him, my boys.

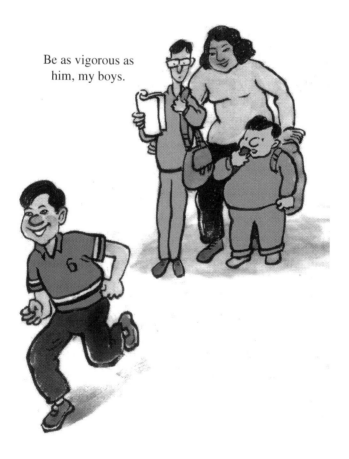

In the United States, Japan and other countries, the same problem has happened in the 1980s. The physical fitness of teenagers has declined along with the improvement of living standards and nutritional status. The countermeasure is to carry out a national program to improve physical fitness. At present, we mainly consider the case from the perspective of sports, such as improving sports facilities and requiring people to do one hour of exercise everyday. I don't believe these measures can fundamentally solve the problem. We should first consider what the main reason for the decline of teenagers' physical fitness is, and then solve it accordingly.

In my opinion, the main reason for the decline of teenagers' physical fitness is the orientation of education. Our main criterion for measuring students is scores, and what lie behind scores are reading, a lot of homework and memory training. It seems like other aspects of a student are not as important. He/she is only required to study well and get high scores. From childhood to adulthood, students devote most of their energy and time to studying. As an extension of the above phenomenon, the surrounding environment, especially parents, is most concerned about their children's intelligence, their ranking and scores in the class, and whether they can go to the university. In such an environment, it is very difficult for a parent to seriously consider the child's physical condition and he/she often feels that if there is no disease, it is OK to make do. However, "physical fitness" and "health" are two different things. It is absolutely unacceptable to define "health" only as not being ill for teenagers. Because the body has greater compensatory ability when people are young, and the decline of heart and lung function is not apparent. The crucial factor in improving the health of teenagers is to increase their physical fitness, including the most important aspects which are muscle strength, heart and lung, and nervous system function. Improving physical fitness is the real way to improve the health of teenagers. The kind of education system with scores and examinations as the core will never improve students' physical fitness.

The change in lifestyle is also an important reason for the decline of teenagers' physical fitness. When I was in primary school, it was very luxurious to ride a bicycle, and I usually walked. The best leisure activity was to watch movies. Entertainment revolved around sports or activities, like singing and acting.

There have been considerable changes in lifestyles since the time of my youth. First, the means of transportation have greatly improved. Many more people travel around by car. Second, computers and the Internet have entered our lives. Data show that computers and the Internet account for 36.2% of students' spare time. Lack of physical activities has led to the decline in students' physical fitness.

I used to engage in competitive sports, which is different from physical exercise. In addition to pursuing exercise of the body, competitive sports also focus on developing willpower, teamwork and high efficiency. I ran the 400m hurdles. On the sporting field, sometimes one has to train for a year to improve the results by one second. The mindset of a race against time, I developed as a result of running has also inspired my work: I am conscious that I should not waste time but improve efficiency. For the majority of young people, actively participating in sports activities, especially competitive sports, can be a shortcut to improving their physical fitness fundamentally. Competitive sports have many benefits. They help develop muscle ability, and heart and lung function. More importantly, through participating in competitive sports, people can imporve their mental health through sublimation.

The top priority is not to choose which way to exercise, but to begin to exercise first. Only with good physical conditions can young students do more work and bear more pressure in the future. Teenagers tend not to understand this point. Why? They are growing and do not feel too many physical problems. They do not care if they are a bit heavy or have relatively high blood pressure. However, when they reach middle age and old age, they will strongly feel the impact of these problems.

"If the youth is strong, our country will be strong." It can be said that improving the physical health of teenagers is a project of significance for the future. At present, the rapid increase of overweight and obese children and adolescents in our nation, as well as the declining trend of physical health, is likely to become a major health hazard for the young and middle-aged labor force in 10 years. The hidden danger to children is also a hidden danger to the future of the nation. The physical fitness of teenagers affects the competitiveness of the nation. As chronic diseases have begun to threaten the health of the labor force, how can we not face such problems directly?

Different exercise styles for different ages

It is unlikely for a person to do the same kind of exercise all his life and never get tired. Futhermore, time is ruthless. It is impossible for the elderly to jump up and down as much as when they were young and bear the same amount of exercise.

Therefore, for those who want to exercise by sports, how should they combine and choose the exercise methods suitable for them at different stages of life? A training expert in the United States recently designed a fitness program that can benefit people for a lifetime. This program helps health-conscious people find suitable exercise methods from their twenties to sixties. The following is the specific plan designed by this training expert for your reference.

20 years old and above: They can choose high impact aerobic exercise like running or boxing. For the body at this stage, these sports have many benefits. They can consume a lot of energy, strengthen the muscles of the whole body, and improve energy level, endurance and hand–eye coordination. Psychologically, these exercises can help people relieve external pressure, temporarily forget daily chores and obtain a sense of accomplishment. At the same time, running has the advantages of stimulating creativity and training self-discipline. Boxing is more suitable to be considered as a "tool for releasing pressure" besides cultivating confidence, continence and coping ability in the face of conflicts.

30 years old and above: It is recommended that they choose rock climbing, skateboarding, skating or martial arts to keep fit. In addition to aiding weight loss, these exercises can strengthen muscle elasticity, especially in hips and legs. They also contribute to vitality and endurance and can improve people's sense of balance, coordination and sensitivity. Psychologically, rock climbing can cultivate meditative concentration and help people build self-confidence and improve strategic thinking. Skating is pleasant, and makes people forget unhappiness. Martial arts help people stay calm, unyielding and vigilent in conflicts, and can also effectively improve the degree of concentration.

40 years old and above: People around this age should choose low impact aerobic exercise, like hiking, climbing stairs, and tennis.

These exercises can increase endurance and strengthen the muscles of the lower body, especially the legs. Exercises such as climbing stairs not only make people sweat and keep fit, but are also suitable for busy office workers to practice conveniently everyday. Tennis is a proper whole-body exercise, which can increase the agility and coordination of various parts of the body and keep people energetic. Meanwhile, the pressure on joints will not be as great as running and high impact aerobic exercise. Psychologically, these exercises can make people feel refreshed, reduce tension and release pressure. Take climbing stairs as an example. Climbing up and down is an excellent way for a person to regain control of himself and restore stability of mood. Similarly, playing tennis has social functions, enables people to put aside pressure and distractions and train their concentration ability, judgment and sense of timing.

50 years old and above: Suitable sports include swimming, weight training, rowing, playing golf, etc. Swimming can effectively strengthen the muscles and enhance the elasticity of all parts of the body. Besides, due to the buoyancy of the water, swimming is not as difficult as land sports. It is especially suitable for convalescents, pregnant women, rheumatic patients and older people. Weight training can make muscles firm, improve bone density and enhance abilities for other exercises. When playing golf, if people can walk on their own, carry their bags and speed up the pace, it will often produce the effect of stabilizing heart function. Psychologically, swimming has both inspiring and calming effects, and concentrating on rowing makes people forget chores. Weight training helps to improve the satisfaction of self-image, allowing stress and irritability to be released with sweat. Rowing in a team can cultivate cooperative ability and team spirit. Playing golf can make people more focused and self-disciplined.

60 years old and above: They should do more walking, ballroom dancing, yoga or aerobic exercise in water. Walking can strengthen both legs and help prevent osteoporosis and joint tension. Ballroom dancing can enhance the sense of rhythm, coordination and elegance of a person. It fits people who do not exercise often. Yoga can make the entire body more elastic and balanced and prevent physical injuries. Aerobic exercise in water mainly enhances muscle strength and body elasticity and is good for the obese, pregnant women or the elderly and the weak.

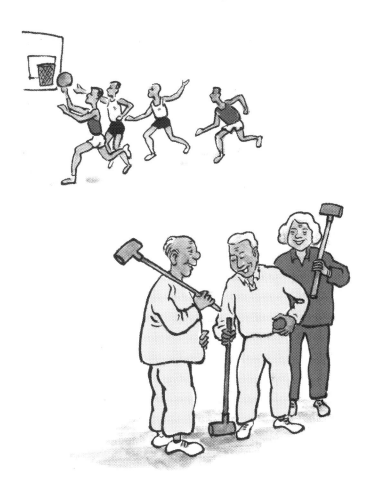

These are not strenuous exercises. Apart from increasing fitness, their greatest function is to help people feel energetic, have fun and remain social. They are a good way for the elderly to retain a young mentality.

Nowadays, many people say that they do not have time to exercise. My advice is to regard physical exercise and functional exercise as indispensable and important components of life, just like eating, working and sleeping, in doing so, your spiritual level will reach a new height and you can find time to exercise. Everyone eats and sleeps no matter whether they have time or not.

It should be the same for the exercise. Without such a mentality, there will never be time. Exercise should be regarded as a conscious act. I hope everyone can realize the truth lying within this point, and start thinking about it now instead of waiting until they get old.

If a person pays attention to the four cornerstones of the health, which are psychological balance, reasonable diet, quitting smoking and limiting alcohol, and proper exercise, then he/she can reduce the probability of high blood pressure by 55%, diabetes by 50%, cerebral infarction by 75% and tumor by 33%.

The next part is the fifth cornerstone of health: early prevention and treatment.

Early prevention and treatment

Human health is like the maintenance of a dam. When leakage has been found at the beginning, it takes limited effort to deal with it. If we do not pay attention and do not fix it until it collapses, even more manpower and material resources spent would not be able to recover it.

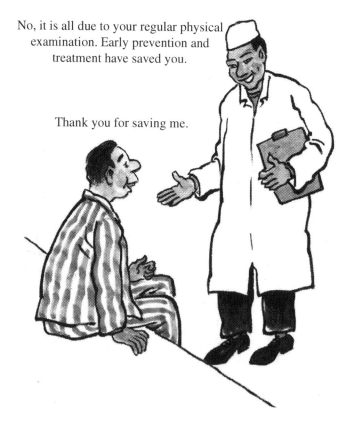

No, it is all due to your regular physical examination. Early prevention and treatment have saved you.

Thank you for saving me.

Minor problems deserve close attention

Yan Xiangrong, a well-known lawyer in Guangzhou, died suddenly in mid-speech. Guo Yu, a brain surgeon from Guangdong Provincial People's Hospital, died suddenly before a complicated surgery... In fact, they had both felt a little bit uncomfortable for some time before the incidents, with symptoms of chest oppression and heart discomfort. However, they didn't take them seriously, and paid with their lives. There are too many examples like them, and many of them were social elites. The phenomenon of "karoshi", which once exclusively characterized the Japanese, has now become common to us.

Not to leave the front line on account of minor wounds is a well-known and inspirational slogan of the Chinese people, and "no pain no gain" is also a life creed believed by many people. These sonorous and passionate slogans have been inspiring people from all areas of life for many years. Many of these people have spared no effort to shed blood and sweat for their work, working hard even if they were ill. They never stopped until the last minute. As a result, we have many role models and touching stories. However, we should perhaps reflect on these and ask, how many outstanding social elites have left us too early and regretfully because of their long-term "minor injuries" and accumulated illness? As a Chinese proverb goes, with the skin gone, to what can the hair attach itself?

Therefore, I suggest that minor problems deserve close attention when there are no emergencies. We should be kind to ourselves in daily life, seek medical treatment in time if we are ill, and stay healthy. It is a pity that I often could not do it myself when was youger. But after SARS, there was something wrong with my body, so now I also pay close attention to my health. The incident has taught me a lesson: people who are busy with their work often ignore minor physical problems, but in fact it is not worthwhile to spend the treatment time on work.

There is a saying, "Human health is like the maintenance of a dam. When leakage has been found at the beginning, it takes limited effort to deal with it. If we do not pay attention and do not fix it until it collapses, even more manpower and material resources spent would not be able to recover it." This saying is valuable and everyone should seriously heed it.

In China, the top 10 diseases, such as tumor, high blood pressure, diabetes, coronary disease, chronic obstructive pulmonary disease, generally start with some small index abnormalities. It often takes 5, 10 or even 15 years before they slowly develop into fatal problems such as myocardial infarction and cerebrovascular accidents. Li Yuanyuan died of cervical cancer at the age of 41, but cervical cancer is actually the only cancer that can be prevented, and the therapeutic effect of early discovery is ideal. Tang Junnian, the 56-year-old former boss of Shanghai Tomson Group, died of diabetic ketoacidosis. We should know that it is a severe diabetic complication that will not happen if only a little attention is paid to the treatment.

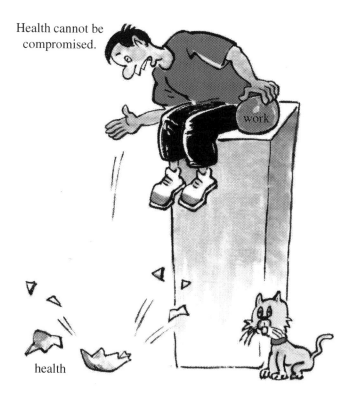

Health cannot be compromised.

health

Gao Xiumin, Fu Biao and others are all familiar social elites who died early in middle age due to diseases of one kind or another. In these cases of premature death, many young and middle-aged people thought that they were young and in good health while ignoring their health issues. They often did not pay much attention to abnormal physical conditions and just lived with them. They did not go to the hospital until the problems became severe. What could originally have been a minor problem if treated early was treated only when it became worse and could not be reversed.

Personally, I believe the difference between health and work is that health is a one-way street: returning to good health from a condition of poor health is very difficult. Health is like a hollow glass ball that will be shattered and gone once it falls to the ground. Work is like a rubber ball, which can bounce up after falling. Life is limited, and health is priceless. Having health does not mean owning everything, but without health, there is nothing. Therefore, I sincerely hope that everyone will cherish their health, pay attention to early prevention and treatment and take care of minor health problems.

Extreme fatigue leads only to death

A survey shows that the numbers of intellectuals dying from overwork in China have been increasing year by year. According to the statistics by the National Bureau of Statistics in 2002, our average life expectancy has increased to 72 years, but the average life expectancy of Chinese intellectuals is only 58 years. The average age of middle-aged senior intellectuals in Zhongguancun is 53 years, in comparison to 58 years decade ago. The survey also found that 3,000 middle-aged intellectuals died in Shenzhen in the past 10 years, with an average age of only 51. This is true in Shenzhen, Beijing, Shanghai and Guangzhou. The phenomenon of premature death is more common among people who work hard and have more achievements. The reason behind it is extreme fatigue. As a proverb goes: "Before the age of 40, one fights for money with his/her life, and after 40, one will buy his/her life with money." I often meet this kind of patients in the hospital, and I have deeply felt the meaning of that saying.

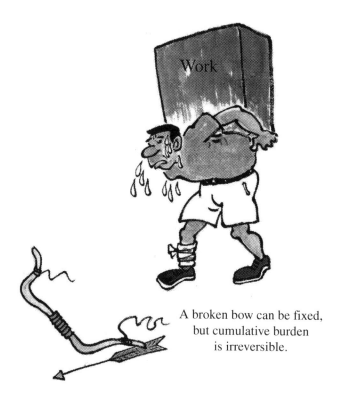

A broken bow can be fixed,
but cumulative burden
is irreversible.

The president of Sun Yat-sen University Cancer Hospital once told me this story. A successful entrepreneur went to their hospital for examination. It was a tumor, but it was discovered too late. The successful entrepreneur said, "I can give as much money as you want, even billions, as long as you can hire the best experts and apply the best technology." But his doctor repiled, "There is nothing I can do. Nobody in the world can fix it. The development of medicine has not yet reached this level — as long as you have the money, you can cure any disease." Why is this happening? It is because we have not paid heed to early prevention and treatment. As we all know, a person can live three times as long as others, but he/she can only live once. Since the beginning of human existence, the number of people who are alive in the world at any point in time is smaller when compared to those who are dead. So, now it is our generation that is alive. How can we live better? Because after a few decades, we will all be gone, and there will be the next generation. There will always be more dead people than living people. It is a natural law. A person is like gurgling water after his/her birth, which needs to be cared for. After passing through mountain springs, he/she will spread the youthful sense. Then he/she will pass through surging rivers, which is the time to give full play to his/her talents. Finally, he/she will flow into the sea quietly. This is the way a person lives, and it will always be. But why do some people live better than others?

Deng Tietao was a famous and senior doctor of traditional Chinese medicine in Guangzhou. Whilst he was over 90 years old, I often cooperated with him to study severe cases of myasthenia. Deng Tietao was good at treating cardiovascular disease. Although he suffered from coronary disease, his speech was full of passion. What is his way of staying in good health? "Pay attention to nourish the mind, regulate the seven emotions, cherish the essence and qi, restrict the appetite, protect the spleen and stomach, eat well, and pay attention to exercise and never overdo anything". I often communicated with Deng Tietao. He asked me what kind of sports I played and I said basketball. He said that playing basketball has too much impact on the body and I should stop playing and do some other suitable sports instead. He created a set of health-preserving methods. He would massage himself and he also practiced health qi gong: Wu Qin Xi, Ba Duan Jin, etc.

Another example is the well-known general General Lv Zhengcao. When he was 101 years old, and looking back on his first 100 years he said, "In my whole life, I have been fighting the Japanese, managing railways and playing tennis". His motto in life is: what matters in life is not how long one lives but how much one has done. Why is he able to live longer than others? The key is understanding the rhythm of life and balanced work and rest.

Ba Jin said, "Beautiful middle-age is a mature period in life. For people in this period, life is as broad as the sea and sky, and they are free to go anywhere they want." The person who cares for you most should be yourself, not a doctor or anyone else. I hope everyone can care for themselves, and live vigorously and happily until they are 70, 80, and 90. Don't become incomplete in terms of health by the age of 50, which will be meaningless.

So, why should we advocate early prevention and treatment?

Early prevention and treatment provide a big return on a small investment

Generally speaking, people who pay more attention to health are older people. If time can be moved backwards 20 to 30 years and prevention is valued when people are in good health, they would have the maximum return with the minimum investment. Clinically, we have carried out health education campaigns over the years to provide self-management information for in-patients of asthma and help them learn self-management techniques. As a result, the recurrence rate of asthma has been reduced by 75%, hospitalization time has been reduced by 54%, and the economic and psychological burden of patients have been greatly decreased.

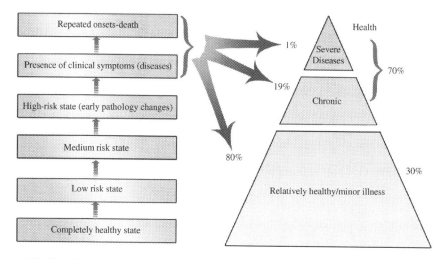

The Correlation between Sketch of Disease Development Process and Medical Expenses.

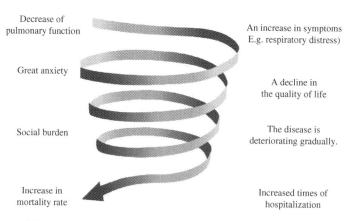

Diagram of the Influences of Deterioration of Disease on Patients.

The least healthy 1% of the population and the 19% suffering from chronic disease share 70% of the medical and health expenses.

The healthiest 70% of the population only spend 10% of the medical and health expenses.

We cannot guarantee that we will always be healthy. Everyone has the probability of becoming the unhealthiest 1% or the 19% suffering from chronic disease. However, we are the masters of our health. We should conduct physical examinations regularly to achieve early detection, early diagnosis and early treatment so as to control any disease in its infancy.

Diseases that people do not feel at early stages of morbidity include:

1. Hyperlipidemia, fatty liver.
2. High blood pressure.
3. Coronary disease.
4. Diabetes.
5. Chronic obstructive pulmonary disease.
6. Tumor.
......

Let me take chronic obstructive pulmonary disease as an example to illustrate the importance of early prevention and treatment. Chronic obstructive pulmonary disease (COPD) is a destructive lung disease. Its symptoms are limited airflow, shortness of breath, cough, asthma and sputum production, which will gradually weaken patients' respiratory function. It has a high morbidity and tends to recur. It has a long course which is progressive and has many complications. People with COPD have to bear with high treatment cost and poor prognosis. The patients often die of respiratory failure and pulmonary heart disease. COPD is currently the fifth leading cause of death in the world, ranking third in China, and showing a progressive upward trend in the world.

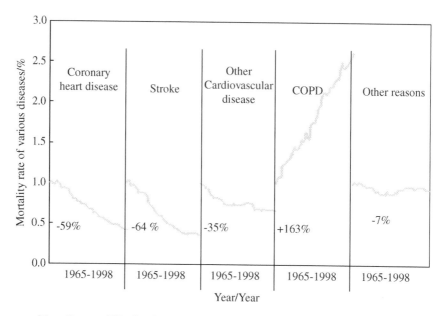

Mortality rate (%) of various diseases in the United States from 1965 to 1998.

In 2007, the results of our survey in nine major cities in the nation showed that the prevalence rate of COPD among people over 40 years old reached 8.2%, of which 12.4% were men and 5.1% were women. It has indicated that there are about 38 million COPD patients nationwide. Theoretically, early detection and treatment can slow down the developing process of COPD, prevent damage to lung tissue, improve the quality of life and reduce the risk of death. However, the early symptoms of COPD are not apparent, and the disease progression is relatively slow. Thus, doctors and patients usually do not pay attention to it, which delays diagnosis and treatment. Our survey has found that about half of the patients were not aware of their illness at all, and the diagnosis rate of doctors was also very low — less than 40%.

For most patients, lung function has already begun to decline before the symptoms appear. This is because many organs of people have strong physiological compensation ability. Some functions of organs can degenerate by about 30% before people's lives are greatly affected. Once the decrease reaches 40% or more, functional losses will multiply, and many problems will be exposed. Therefore, by the time some people found themselves climbing stairs with shortness of breath and walking with respiratory distress, they are already in the middle and late stages of COPD and the best time for treatment had passed. Such episodes would then recur repeatedly, and patients would be hospitalized again and again, which would cost a fortune.

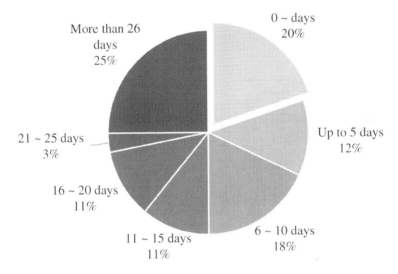

**The number of days of acute attack of COPD in the past 6 months.
(Total number of investigated patients: 752)**

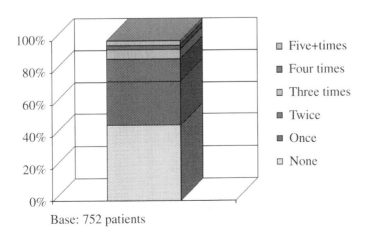

Base: 752 patients

Number of times of hospitalization of COPD patients in one year.

The results of acute exacerbation of COPD in several hospitals participating in the survey has shown that in six months, the number of patients with more than 10 days of acute exacerbation of COPD accounts for 50%. The proportion of patients who need to be hospitalized more than once a year is more than 60%. What a financial burden this disease is.

Therefore, I suggest that the high-risk groups of COPD should be routinely examined. These include people who have been smoking for a long time (especially those over 40 years old who smoke a lot), people who suffer from repeated respiratory tract infection, people who suffer from long-term indoor pollution such as smoke caused by burning firewood in rural areas, and people who are engaged in occupations with dust environments.

Conduct regular physical examination to detect diseases early

Many doctors often hear the same words in clinical practice: "I have always been well. Why did I get so sick so quickly?" High blood pressure, diabetes, coronary disease, tumors, COPD, cerebrovascular accidents and many other chronic disorders generally display no symptoms in the early stage. When typical symptoms occur, they are often in the middle and late stages, thus greatly increasing the difficulty and cost of treatment. Hence, regular physical examination can detect some imperceptible early diseases in a timely manner, and people can then intervene and get them treated as early as possible.

In this way, we can greatly reduce the morbidity rate of chronic disease, disability rate and mortality rate. Due to the popularization of regular physical examination, some advanced countries have effectively controlled the morbidity of chronic diseases. For example, in Germany, 95% of the population have a medical examination once a year. Meanwhile, the high blood pressure morbidity has decreased by 4%, and the coronary disease morbidity by 16%.

The advantage of regular physical examination lies not only in reducing morbidity but also in saving a considerable amount of medical expenses. German economists believe that for every euro invested in physical examination, 3–6 euros can be saved in medical costs. Hong Zhaoguang, a health education expert, has pointed out that for Chinese people, the investment of one yuan in the early physical examination and prevention can save at least eight to nine yuan in medical expenses and 100 yuan in corresponding rescue expenses. In reality, many citizens always feel that regular physical examination requires a large sum of money and are not willing to invest hundreds of yuan to find out about their health status. A survey completed by Fudan School of Public Health has found that the current situation of physical examination of urban residents in China is still not promising. Of the 900 respondents, less than 50% have medical examinations every year, and the awareness of medical examination among males and young people is even weaker.

People who are busier at work, and have more achievements and success in their careers, are also more likely to neglect their health. According to the data from the "Survey on the Health Status of 100 Private Entrepreneurs" in Zhejiang Province, 48% of entrepreneurs admitted that they had not had a comprehensive examination within one year. About 5% relied too much on drugs or doctors, ignoring the regulatory effects of exercise, mindset and other factors. What is more serious is that most entrepreneurs do not know how to relieve pressure and just take on all the pressure, thus creating a huge burden on their bodies. When disease eventually strikes, it is already too late. As a matter of fact, compared with women, men face greater pressure and intensity at work. Many men also have bad living habits such as relatively greater consumption of alcohol and tobacco, more social activities and less exercise. They belong to the population with a high incidence of diseases and should pay more attention to regular physical examination.

At present, 80% of the population who take physical examinations in our nation do so in company physical examination, 10% do so for the purpose of recruitment, and the proportion of individuals who take voluntary physical examination is only 10%. We should widely promote awareness of physical examination in whole society and spread health examination knowledge, so that more and more people will take the initiative to go for regular physical examinations, which provide advanced protection for health.

Advocate personalized health examination

Currently, people who take part in company physical examination form the majority of the "physical examination population" in our nation. However, what is examined in the company physical examination is basically the same for everyone. Practically, people of different age, gender and occupation should have a different emphasis on examination items.

For example, white-collar workers are often in a highly tense mental state, which tends to cause cardiovascular, cervical, lumbar and other conditions. The working environment of those workers also contains "dangers" to their health. They usually work in air-conditioned rooms for long hours and have to face an environment full of computers, making them vulnerable to electromagnetic radiation. Besides, due to long-term desk work, they are prone to "computer syndrome", cervical spondylosis, lumbar spondylosis and other condition over time. Therefore, the physical examination of white-collar workers should pay special attention to the examination for cardiovascular and cerebrovascular diseases, and checks on the cervical vertebrae, lumbar vertebrae and blood.

Middle-aged people often have problems such as high blood pressure, high blood lipids, high blood sugar and low immune function. The probability of these causing cardiovascular and cerebrovascular diseases is extremely high. Therefore, people over 40 years old should care more about the detection of diabetes, high blood pressure, coronary disease, cerebral infarction and some tumors. For some special groups, regular physical examination should be put on the agenda. Specifically, for people in high-risk groups such as those who have been smoking for more than 10 years, they should be more alert as their morbidity of lung cancer has increased significantly. Only with a healthy body can life have true value.

Personalization should be advocated in physical examination. Before the test, it is best to let the physical examination specialist have an understanding of the participant's past medical history, family medical history, physical status, etc. Then the physical examination menu can be set. This is the beginning of an effective physical examination. Personal medical history, especially the medical history of important diseases, is an important reference for doctors performing physical examinations to determine the health status of the participants.

Regular physical examination can prevent minor problems and nip problems in the bud

The occurrence, development and progression of diseases is a natural process. People don't care much about the symptoms at the beginning of many diseases. By the time they feel that the problem is serious, they often have missed the best timing for treatment. In the process of arteriosclerosis in the human body, blood vessels are healthy at first. Then, slowly, some tears are created, which are often due to factors like high blood pressure. What can be used to fill the gaps? Cholesterol. As soon as cholesterol is filled in the gaps, it will gather platelets to form clots. Clots increase over time, and every year blood vessels become

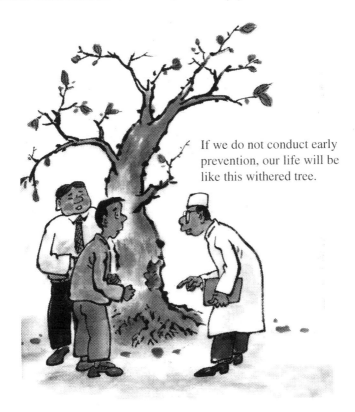

If we do not conduct early prevention, our life will be like this withered tree.

narrower by 1%–2%. If people smoke or have hyperlipidemia, high blood pressure, etc., the speed of vascular stenosis will accelerate to 3%–4%, finally blocking up the blood vessels. This is how coronary disease develops. In fact, there will be signs in the early stage, such as precordial discomfort. If people don't pay attention, small problems eventually end up as myocardial infarction.

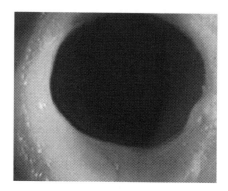

Sectional view of a 50% clogged blood vessel.

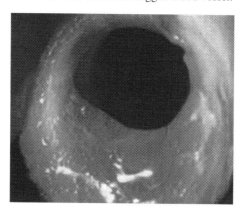

Sectional view of a 70% clogged blood vessel.

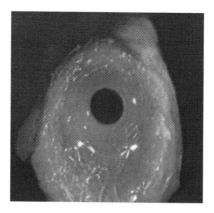

Sectional view of a 90% clogged blood vessel.
Sectional views of human blood vessels — Different Periods and Shapes.

When blood vessels are clogged by 50%, a person may have no feeling of discomfort; if they are 70% clogged, dizziness and numbness of hands and feet may be felt; once they are clogged by 90%, stroke and hemiplegia (paralysis on one side of the body) may occur at any time.

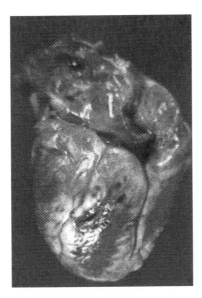

Rupture of the heart.

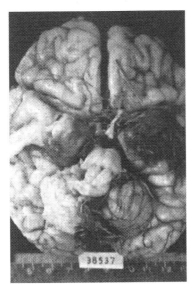

Cerebral hemorrhage caused by the rupture of cerebral vessels.

The same is true for cerebral vessels. At first, they are unobstructed. When people have an unbalanced diet, their cholesterol level increase over time, and they develop hyperlipidemia. Slowly, some cholesterol plaques will adhere to the vessel walls, and platelets will gather, which will gradually make the blood vessel narrower. At this time, there may not be any symptoms. When the stenosis reaches a certain level, the consequence will be cerebral apoplexy (bleeding within the brain), and the difficulty of treatment is huge.

Famous actor Gu Yue died of extensive myocardial infarction. Famous sketch comedy actor Gao Xiumin died of sudden myocardial infarction. Just imagine, if they had received regular physical examinations, paid attention to the revealed information that is, early detection and early prevention and also received early treatment, they might not have died so early. If outstanding elites can live an average of another 10 to 20 years, will they not make greater contributions to the nation?

Most cancers can be cured if discovered early

In the eyes of many people, cancer (malignant tumor) is seen as an incurable disease. Cancer is indeed dangerous, but it is not that lethal nor a cause of inevitable death as depicted in some movies and novels. Lots of data have proven that cancer is a "treatable disease." According to domestic and foreign reports, the five-year recovery rate (except for liver cancer) in early-stage cancer is above 90%. If the cases of early-stage cancer and late-stage cancer are added together, the five-year recovery rate of the 10 major cancers also reaches 41%. As a head scientist in charge of tumor research in the United States once said, "We often hear that cancer is the most feared disease in the United States, but what is surprising is that it is one of the chronic diseases with the best recovery rate in the nation." There is no doubt that we are not in a very optimistic situation, because, as mentioned above, the recovery rate of early-stage cancer can be up to 90%, while the combined recovery rate of early-stage cancer and late-stage cancer is only about 40%, with a difference of 60%. Therefore, the key to improving cancer's recovery rate lies in early detection, diagnosis and treatment.

Dr. Rickenbacker, head of the National Cancer Institute of the United States, said that progress in biomedical technology has made detection methods more effective and treatment technology more advanced. It lets cancer be found and treated early, and greatly reduces cancer's mortality rate.

Take lung cancer as an example. Because of factors such as air pollution in the environment and the continuous rise of the number of smokers, the prevalence rate of lung cancer has been continuously increasing in recent decades. In the past 20 years, the mortality rate of lung cancer in China has gone up significantly for both men and women. From 1973 to 1992, the mortality rate of lung cancer in China increased by 158%–194% for men and 122.55% for women. For instance, in Shanghai, Beijing and other big cities, male patients have always been far ahead in the morbidity rate of lung cancer and are firmly in the first place. Among women with cancer, although breast cancer ranks first, lung cancer has come from behind and risen to the second and third positions. The mortality rate of lung cancer in both men and women has already taken first place in Shanghai. In 2002, the number of new lung cancer cases in China was 269,650, ranking first among all new tumor cases in that year. Meanwhile, the number of lung cancer deaths was 340,360, ranking first too. However, the therapeutic effectiveness in treating lung cancer has not increased significantly in the past 10 years. The five-year survival rate is only 10%–15%, and the cost of hospitalization for advanced lung cancer is also very high.

Take 38 cases of adenocarcinoma (cancer beginning in glandular cells) and 74 cases of squamous cell carcinoma (skin cancer) in 1998 as examples. The average hospitalization cost per person per admission (medical expenses, treatment expenses, operation expenses, examination expenses, laboratory expenses, radiotherapy expenses, blood transfusion expenses and other expenses) was 18019.44 yuan for patients in stage I, 26186.74 yuan for patients in stage II, 22006.40 yuan for patients in stage III and 32534.10 yuan for patients in stage IV.

The study found that although the five-year survival rate of stage I lung cancer can reach more than 80%, unfortunately, there were too few diagnoses for early lung cancer. 80% of lung cancer patients were in the late stage at the time of diagnosis, and the proportion of early diagnosis only accounted for 5% of advanced lung cancer patients. Therefore, early detection and treatment are very important!

Our research institute cooperated with Zhuhai Health Care Office to carry out cancer screening tests for local officials. In 1994, we began to use low-dose spiral CT (the radiation dose of this method is only one-sixth of that of normal CT and has less impact on the human body) to carry out screening work on 460 high-risk groups. By 2002, a total of 4,400 people had been surveyed annually for a total of 8 years, and 48 cases of lung cancer and 32 cases of other benign lesions had been detected.

Selection criteria for high-risk group of lung cancer:

1. The respondent is above 45–50 years old.
2. The respondent has a smoking history of more than 10 years.
3. The respondent has a family history of tumor or the respondent him/herself has a history of tumor or tuberculosis.
4. The respondent has a history of contact with occupational or environmental pollution.

Among the above 48 cases of lung cancer patients, 36 cases had masses smaller than 1.5 cm, 8 cases were stage II, and 4 cases were stage III, with a detection rate of 1.04%. The five-year survival rate of stage I lung cancer after minimally invasive and radical surgery was 85%. It is known that the five-year survival rate of lung cancer is very low and generally at only 15%. However, in our study, the five-year survival rate of lung cancer was greatly improved to 85% due to the general survey, which enabled early detection of tumors and early treatment. What a surprising result!

In the case of one patient, CT found a small tumor in his lung during physical examination. After an expert consultation, it was decided that surgery should be performed. As a result, adenocarcinoma was removed. Because it was at the early stage, he is still in good spirits and living well now. If early detection had not occured at the beginning, the tumor would have grown and metastasized after one year. By then it would have been hopeless for the patient. Sometimes it is just that close.

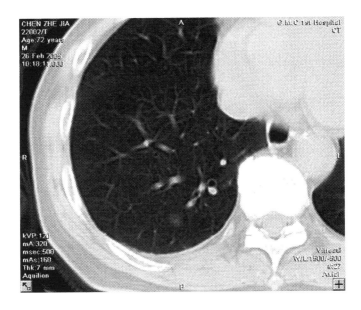

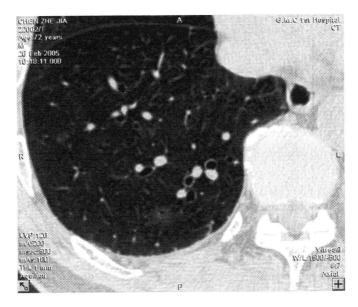

7 mm ground glass-like nodule shadow. From 1 mm thick scan we can clearly observe small cavity lesions in the nodule, which was confirmed by surgery as alveolar carcinoma.

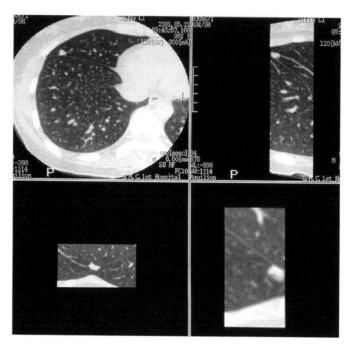

Small adenocarcinoma, observation from multiple levels.

Another recent large-scale multi-center study has further confirmed the importance of early detection. The study examined 31,567 asymptomatic people with a smoking history, a history of occupational exposure, or a history of secondhand smoke exposure. It then evaluated the 10-year survival rate of those with stage I lung cancer within the whole group. Of the total population that received screening, 484 were diagnosed with lung cancer, and 412 were in phase I (85%). The 10-year survival rate of these patients with stage I lung cancer was 88%. 302 of them underwent surgery within one month after diagnosis, and their 10-year survival rate increased to 92%. 8 patients did not receive treatment and were all dead within 5 years after diagnosis. The researcher Dr. Horovitz said,

> If it is stage I lung cancer, the 10-year survival rate will be 88%. The simplest way to find stage I lung cancer is spiral CT. If you can diagnose early, although you cannot be sure of how long they will live, you definitely can let them live for 10 more years. However, this can be very difficult to achieve if patients come to seek medical treatment and diagnosis after clinical symptoms have occurred. Besides, the operation cost for stage I lung cancer is less than half of the treatment cost for advanced lung cancer.

The results of this study captured attention in the medical field. Dr. Robert Smith, director of cancer screening at the American Cancer Society, said, "This discovery is of great significance. It comes from multiple centers. This screening method can be successfully applied to other situations." Dr. Len Horovitz, a lung specialist at Lenox Hill Hospital in New York City, said, "This is an essential discovery. If you can find lung cancer at an early stage, it can be said that you can cure it. Lung cancer is the number one killer, but diagnosis often comes out too late."

Therefore, a physical examination once a year can help reveal many problems at an early stage, such as lung cancer, liver cancer, gastric cancer, intestinal cancer, breast cancer, cervical cancer, and prostate cancer.

The same is true for liver cancer. Small liver cancer can be detected by ordinary ultrasound scan. After the operation is done and the cancer is removed, the prognosis will be much better.

The case of prostate cancer is also similar. Studies have found that prostate cancer can increase the level of a kind of prostate-specific antigen (PSA) in patients. Examining the change of PSA in the body is helpful for the detection of the onset of prostate cancer. It can improve the early diagnosis rate of prostate cancer.

Gynecological tumors are not uncommon now, especially cervical cancer, which ranks first in terms of morbidity. There are about 450,000 new cases worldwide every year, 80% of which occur in developing countries. Every year, 20,000 to 30,000 women worldwide die of cervical cancer.

Because of the extensive development of general screening and treatment in China, morbidity and mortality rate of cervical cancer have decreased significantly. The mortality rate was 10.28/(100,000) in the 1970s, and 3.25/(100,000) in the 1990s, a decrease by 68.4%. The morbidity rate in China's developed cities has reached the lowest level in the world. However, in recent years, due to the significant growth in the infection rate of human papillomavirus (HPV), the onset of cervical cancer has shown signs of a rebound and tends to affect more young people.

However, although cervical cancer is the most common cause of malignant tumor in gynecology, it is also the only preventable gynecological cancer. Therefore, when women reach a certain age and do a very simple cytological examination and virus detection every year, they can detect, deal with and solve the problem early.

Save more breasts

Breast cancer is also a major problem. The American Cancer Society has estimated that 182,000 new breast cancer patients were found in the United States in 1994, and about 46,000 women died of breast cancer which ranked first in gynecological cancer. In China, the number of new breast cancer patients is also rising rapidly. The reason is yet to be clarified, but it may be related to lifestyle and diet. From 1994 to 2003 in Guangzhou, 288,857 cases of breast diseases were monitored, and the average detection rate of proliferation of mammary gland was

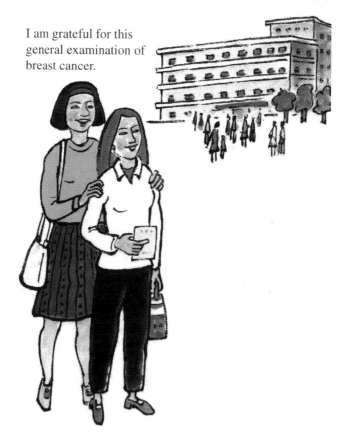

I am grateful for this general examination of breast cancer.

49.3/(100,000). The detection rate of breast cancer reached 123.7/(100,000) in 2003. The most vulnerable age group was 40–49 years old.

In Shanghai, from 1972 to 1974, the detection rate of breast cancer was 18.3/(100,000), and from 1987 to 1989, 25.1/(100,000), an increase of 37.6%.

In Beijing, from 1990 to 1991, the detection rate of breast cancer was 25.7/(100,000), and in 2000, 35.1/(100,000), an increase of 36.6%.

Therefore, I very much agree with my friend Professor Xu Guangwei's national breast cancer screening campaign for one million women. Breast cancer is fairly easy to detect and prevent, and the procedures of treatment are not complicated. Radical mastectomy is not necessarily needed when breast cancer is found. In many cases, removing the lesions and treatment is sufficient to solve the problem. These examinations should be kept in mind especially by women over 40 years old, those who are not pregnant, those who have not breast-fed or have a family history of breast cancer, or those who have had many years of benign lesions. Women should learn to do self-examination and spend 15 minutes everyday to self-examine and maintain their health.

Early warning signs of common cancer

Many books, magazines or websites about cancer and health in our nation provide information on early detection of cancer. Here are some of them. You can refer to relevant books for details.

A. Eight warning signs
The WHO once put forward the following "eight warning signs" as a reference for people to detect early-stage cancer.

(1) Hard lump (induration), such as hard lumps found in breast, under the skin or on tongue.
(2) Obvious change in warts (excrescences) or moles.
(3) Persistent digestive disorder.
(4) Persistent hoarseness, dry cough and dysphagia (difficulties in swallowing).
(5) Menstrual disorder, a massive amount of menstrual bleeding, and bleeding outside the usual monthly period.

(6) Unexplained bleeding in nose, ear, bladder or intestinal tract.
(7) Wounds or swelling which do not heal.
(8) Weight loss for unknown causes.

B. Ten major symptoms
Based on the situation in our country, the Chinese Academy of Medical Sciences has proposed the following ten symptoms as warning signs to alert people of tumors.

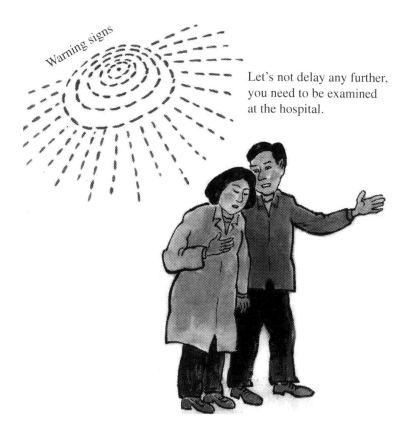

Warning signs

Let's not delay any further, you need to be examined at the hospital.

(1) A lump in any part of the body, such as the breast, neck, or abdomen, especially a gradually growing one.
(2) Ulcers not caused by injuries in any part of the body, such as the tongue, buccal mucosa (check lining and back of month), skin, etc., especially those that do not heal for a long time.

(3) Irregular vaginal bleeding or secretions (commonly known as leucorrhea) of women over middle age.

(4) Substernal pain, burning pain, or foreign body sensation after eating or progressive aggravation of dysphagia.

(5) Dry cough that cannot be cured for a long time or blood in sputum.

(6) Long-term dyspepsia, progressive anorexia, emaciation, no apparent causes.

(7) Changes in bowel habits or hematochezia (fresh blood in stools).

(8) Nasal congestion, nose bleeds, unilateral headache (on one side) or double vision.

(9) Sudden growth or ulceration, bleeding of the mole, or fall off of the original hair on the mole.

(10) Painless hematuria (blood in urine).

In addition to the above eight warning signs and ten major symptoms, the following signs should also be taken into serious consideration.

(1) Unilateral persistent aggravation of headache, vomiting and vision disorder, especially diplopia of unknown causes.

(2) Tinnitus, hearing loss, blood from the nose which appears in sputum, or neck lump.

(3) Unexplained oral bleeding, discomfort in the part of the throat behind the mouth, foreign body sensation or oral pain.

(4) Painless and continuously aggravating jaundice.

(5) Nipple discharge, especially bloody fluid.

(6) Enlargement of breast tissue in males.

(7) Unexplained fatigue, anemia and fever.

(8) Unexplained systemic pain, bone and joint pain.

Additionally, precancerous lesions should also be regarded as early signs. Lesions like mucosal leukoplakia (white/grey patches in the mouth), chronic ulcer of skin, fistula, proliferative scar (especially scar caused by chemical burns), atrophic gastritis (inflammation of stomach lining) and intestinal metaplasia (transformation of upper digestive tract cells into intestine-like cells), multiple polyps of the rectum, keratosis (especially in the haad muscles), cystic hyperplasia of the breast (breast cysts), cervical erosion (development of cervical cells outside the cervix), and cervical polyps can develop into cancer.

C. Deal with early signs properly

It must be stressed that neither the eight warning signs nor any of the ten symptoms are exclusive to cancer. Having one or even several of these symptoms does not necessarily mean one has developed cancer. For example, some pulmonary fungal infections or granulomatous diseases of the lung have symptoms of cough and hemoptysis (coughing up of blood). The chest radiographs or CT also resemble lung cancer, but they are not lung cancer. Vaginal fungal infections of endometrial proliferation which are common among middle-aged women can also lead to massive menstrual bleeding and leucorrhea. Esophagitis (inflammation of tube carring food to stomach) and esophageal diverticulum (abnormal development of pouch in the esophagus lining) can also cause substernal pain, discomfort and burning pain after eating. Patients with chronic atrophic gastritis often suffer from dyspepsia and anorexia. Ulcerative colitis (colon/rectum inflammation and ulcers) and intestinal polyps can also cause hematochezia. Nasal polyps and migraine can also cause unilateral nasal congestion and headache. In schistosomiasis endemic areas, chylous hematuria ("milky" urine with blood) can also be caused by parasites.

In short, having one or several of the above warning signs or symptoms is not equivalent to suffering from cancer. These signs cannot be regarded as the basis for the diagnosis of cancer. They should never be the reason for panic and anxiety in the family. However, the above warning signs and symptoms may indeed belong to some early signs of cancer. If these signs are taken lightly, diagnosis and treatment will often be delayed.

D. Early signs of common cancer

(1) Esophageal cancer: Feeling of slowness, retention or slight choking when swallowing food, which can subside on its own, but appear again after a few days, recurring and gradually aggravating. Pain in sternum when swallowing saliva or eating. Foreign body sensation in the esophagus, which is not caused by eating and persists, does not subside after drinking water nor swallowing food.

(2) Gastric cancer: Sudden occurrence of dyspepsia symptoms of unknown causes that persist and progress rapidly. The prominent manifestations are the rapid loss of appetite, abdominal fullness

and discomfort after eating, and evident weight loss at the same time. Alternately, people who did not have stomachache ("heart pain") in the past suddenly suffer from repeated stomachache. For people who have had stomachache before, a sudden and recent change in the intensity, nature and onset time of the pain to the extent that the drugs that were originally effective for treatment become ineffective or less effective.

(3)   Colorectal cancer: The possibility of colorectal cancer should be considered for people over 30 years old who suffer from abdominal discomfort, dull pain, abdominal distension, changes in bowel habits, constipation or diarrhea or occurrence of them in turns, dragging sensation, bloody stool, anemia, fatigue and weakness, and abdominal lumps. Localized and intermittent dull pain along the colon is the first warning signal for colon cancer. Obvious feeling of dragging with blood in stool is a signal of rectal cancer (colorectal cancer includes colon cancer and rectal cancer).

(4)   Liver cancer: Early liver cancer shows no specific symptoms, and most of the common symptoms are some complicated manifestations of precancerous diseases. However, if patients with chronic hepatitis or liver cirrhosis suffer from stabbing or aggravating pain in the right upper abdomen or liver region, physical discomfort, anorexia, progressive dyspepsia, refractory (unresponsive to conventional treament) diarrhea and evident weight loss, they should seek early medical attention.

(5)   Nasopharyngeal Carcinoma (nose cancer): Early signs of nasopharyngeal carcinoma have a common feature, which is that symptoms (and signs) mostly occur on one side. Unilateral bloody snot (blood that is blown out), unilateral nosebleeds, unilateral tinnitus, unilateral hearing loss, unilateral headache, unilateral swelling of lymph nodes in the neck.

(6)   Breast cancer: Abnormal changes in the breast, such as thickening or lumps, swelling, appearance slightly concave ("dimpling sign"), thickening and redness of skin, nipple deformation, retraction or scales, etc. Pain or pressing pain, unilateral nipple discharge in non-lactating women that starts suddenly (lacteal, bloody, or watery liquid).

(7) Cervical cancer: The early symptoms of cervical cancer mainly include the following aspects.
   - Vaginal drip bleeding after sexual intercourse, defecation or urination, of which blood is mixed in vaginal secretions. Discharge appears in small quantity at first and often stops on its own.
   - Irregular vaginal bleeding, especially sudden vaginal bleeding after years of cessation of menstruation.
   - Increased leucorrhea discharge, bloody or pink and watery.
   - Pain in lower abdomen and waist.

   Those who have more than one of the above items should seek early medical advice. Emphasis is placed on irregular vaginal bleeding, contact bleeding and increased leucorrhea discharge.

(8) Brain tumors: They mainly manifest as headache and vomiting. The headache from a brain tumor is often most intense when people wake up in the morning and subsides after that. It is obvious in the forehead, upper neck and back of the head and both sides of the head. The headache is often accompanied by projectile vomit, which has nothing to do with diet, especially when the pain is severe. The headache is relieved after vomiting.

(9) Leukemia: Fever, hemorrhage and anemia are the three early symptoms of (acute) leukemia. The body temperature is between 37.5–38.5°C, and this fever is often accompanied by some form of infection, such as inflammation of skin, in the respiratory tract, intestinal tract, oral cavity, urinary system and other parts of the body. Bleeding can occur anywhere, but common bleeding is subcutaneous, oral, nasal, or in the gums. The degree of bleeding can range from tiny spots and bruises to massive bleeding of the oral and nasal cavity. The anemia is caused by hematopoietic disorder and hemorrhage, progresses rapidly and causes patients to look pale. In addition, swelling of lymph nodes and joint pain may occur, and what is of characteristic meaning is light pressing pain in the sternum.

E. Self-examination

Apart from knowing the above warning signals of cancer, learning to perform self-examination is more conducive to the early detection of cancer.

(1) Check the neck, armpit, and groin for swollen lymph nodes at least once a month (it is generally believed that lymph nodes smaller than the size of a peanut are acceptable). Examine the texture of the swollen lymph nodes and find out whether they are fixed and whether there is pressing pain.

(2) For long-term coughs, attention should be paid to the existence of blood streaks in the sputum, the time of coughing, the location of chest pain, the amount of blood, and the color of the blood.

(3) When there is a loss of appetite, emaciation and epigastric pain, which is accompanied by nausea and vomiting, people should be careful and observe whether there is dark brown content in the vomitus, whether there is black, abnormally foul-smelling or bloody stool, and whether the shape of the stool has changed.

(4) Women should observe whether leucorrhea is mixed with bloody secretions and whether leucorrhea is foul-smelling everyday or every week.

(5) Watch out for changes in bowel and bladder habits. Pay special attention to whether there is pain, dragging feeling and changes in appearance of feces when defecating. When urinating, observe whether the range is shortened, whether there are white secretions discharged, whether there is hematuria, whether there is discomfort in the perineum or anywhere else.

(6) In case of long-term fever with unknown causes, the body temperature should be measured four times a day for three consecutive days, and the results should be recorded. The four times of measurement are in the morning, noon, evening, and at night, respectively. Check blood routine and erythrocyte sedimentation rate when necessary.

(7) Men should be careful if their foreskin is long, pay attention to whether there are ulcers or nodules at the opening of the urethral and whether there are cauliflower-shaped warts that bleed easily in the crown of the penis.

(8) When limb pain occurs, and movement is limited after strenuous activities, people should check to see if their limb joints are swollen and whether there are subcutaneous lumps. If there are painless lumps on the long bones of limbs, people should seek timely medical attention.

(9) Always pay attention to the changes of moles on various parts of the body surface to see if they grow rapidly and ulcerate in a short period of time.

Printed in the United States
by Baker & Taylor Publisher Services